D1245407

BACK IN TIME

Bi†KITCHEN

PALEO - VEGAN YUM!

From

ILLNESS To

BUSINESS

How I reclaimed my health and set
a course to help **YOU** do the same

By Carol McCarthy, MS, CHHC, AADP.

From Illness to Business

Copyright ©2015 by Carol McCarthy

All rights reserved. No part of this book may be reproduced in any form or by any electronic or mechanical means, including information storage and retrieval systems, without permission in writing from the author. For information, contact Carol McCarthy at www.backintimekitchen.com.

The content of this book is for general instruction only. Each person's physical, emotional, and spiritual condition is unique. The instruction in this book is not intended to replace or interrupt the reader's relationship with a physician or other professional. Please consult your doctor for matters pertaining to your specific health and diet.

To contact the author, visit
 www.backintimekitchen.com

ISBN - 10: 0-692-39193-2
ISBN - 13: 978-0-692-39193-8
Printed in the United States of America

"Carol's determination jumps out from every page and it becomes impossible not to share in her passion for nutrition and self-healing. The reader is in a position to benefit from these nuggets of knowledge that Carol so generously offers in this comprehensive look at her personal health journey. An easy read filled with inspiration and hope!!"

~ Jill Perlmutter, Personal Trainer,
Certified Health Coach

"This book is truly inspiring and a "must read" for anyone who wants to achieve a better level of health and wellness in their life, regardless of whether they have medical challenges. It is a book for all of us. I am thankful that Carol was willing to share her knowledge, her wisdom and her empowered life journey in a way that I can immediately apply to my own life."

~ Mary E. Cobb, MS, Business Strategist,
Patient Advocacy Consultant

"I highly recommend this book to anyone suffering with a chronic health issue. Not only is it enjoyable to read her story, but Carol McCarthy offers inspiration and helpful guidance on how to help yourself on a path to full recovery."

~ Susan Blum, MD, MPH
Author, The Immune System Recovery Plan

DEDICATION

For Erin, Keith, and John.
You put the life in my years.

TABLE OF
CONTENTS

DISCLAIMER

I am not a doctor. I was a biochemistry major in college but worked in the field of genetics, not food biochemistry or nutrition. This book is my story and the summary of information that I have gathered along the way. There are some things that I have read so many times that I have come to believe them to be universal truths. They have become part of who I am and what I believe in, scientifically and philosophically. My cumulative knowledge is my interpretation of the many books, magazines, and journals I have read over the past dozen years. If I remembered exactly which book I read a particular fact in, I made sure to mention it specifically in my story. I highly encourage you to read them. You will not regret it. My constant pursuit of knowledge has provided me with many insights. These insights have given me hope, health, and a new life. I firmly believe that no one diet or lifestyle is the answer for everyone. But I hope my story inspires you to find your answers, because I know that it is possible for you to feel better than you do right now.

"I believe in pink. I believe that laughing is the best calorie burner. I believe in kissing, kissing a lot. I believe in being strong when everything seems to be going wrong. I believe that happy girls are the prettiest girls. I believe that tomorrow is another day and I believe in miracles."

—Audrey Hepburn

CHAPTER ONE
MY STORY

Lucky Charms. Mmmmm! I can almost hear the squeak of the chalky marshmallows between my teeth. But, of course, I never started with the marshmallows. First, I poured a huge bowl from the box, then drowned them in skim milk (NEVER whole milk!), and plopped down in front of the TV for several hours of Saturday morning cartoons. There was a method to eating Lucky Charms: First, methodically spoon out all the sugar coated, puffed grain pieces. Second, savor spoonful after spoonful of marshmallow delight. Third, drink the still cold, light greenish-blue milk remaining. Fourth, return to kitchen to refill bowl. I basically started every day of my childhood with a huge bowl of sugary cereal. Captain Crunch, Frosted Flakes (they were GREAT!), Apple Jacks, and my favorite, Quisp: you name it and I scarfed it down. Lunches were primarily made up of cold cut sandwiches on a stale roll if my dad made it (sorry dad). If I was lucky enough to get one of my mom's famous "Scrumptious Sandwiches" then I'd have a carefully layered variety of ham, bologna, and salami, topped with lettuce, tomato and mayo. Dinner was a combination of hotdogs, fried chicken and hamburger helper—burnt, if my dad made it (sorry again, dad!). We did not have a lot of money, so if we ever had the good fortune of going out to eat, it was usually to McDonald's. And I loved it! Well, I could probably tell a thousand stories about the food I grew up on but you get the picture. I grew up eating junk and my dad was not a very good cook. (Dad, maybe you should stop reading my book now!)

I continued these stellar eating habits through high school, college, post grad, and early marriage. I remember taking my toddlers to Wendy's thinking that I was providing them with a healthier choice than McDonald's. Because, of course, I was much more educated than my parents and could afford the upgrade. Until this time, I was a healthy weight and rarely got sick. I remember attending a religious retreat after my first two kids were born. On the retreat, many women shared their life stories and how they came to have a closer relationship with God. The stories were intense. One woman had been raped and one sexually abused by her father.

Yet they turned their pain into an opportunity to become stronger and help others grow in their faith. I remember thinking that I could never give a talk on a retreat because I had had a great life! I was having a devoted love affair with Kellogg's, Oscar Meyer, and the Hamburgler. What could possibly go wrong? I was very unprepared for the kick in the head that was about to come.

A couple of weeks after my third child turned two, I was diagnosed with breast cancer. Although, I have to say, there was a silver lining: a cute, short haircut for the first time in my life, a new wardrobe to fit my size 6 body courtesy of the chemo diet, and endless homemade meals from my friends. Not to mention all the babysitting provided by my mom and in-laws. But I don't think the year I lost to surgery, chemo, and reconstruction was worth the fringe benefits. A scientist at heart, I decided to turn this despicable time period into a learning experience. I read every book, magazine, and scientific journal about cancer that I could find. I became a self-proclaimed expert in the causes of cancer and the conventional and alternative treatments available. I decided then and there that I was not ready to leave this world with a two, four and six year old still left to raise. So, I began to incorporate what I had control over into my lifestyle choices. In short, I became a vegetarian and started exercising several days a week. I could write an entire book about the experience of having cancer—from my amazing oncologist, to the friends who stepped up to the plate for me, and what I learned from all of my subsequent research—but unfortunately (and fortunately!), my story didn't end there.

For years prior to my cancer diagnosis, I had been plagued by pain in my hip joints and neck. At the time of my diagnosis, I had been sleeping sitting up in bed for four years because it was too painful for me to sleep laying down. I had been to countless doctors, none of which could figure out why. But there was no shortage of Cortisone shots, steroids, and anti-inflammatories that they were willing to give me even though they didn't know why I was in pain. Because my oncologist was AWESOME, I asked him if he knew of a doctor that could help me with my back pain. He sent me to a rheumatologist. Genius! It wasn't long before I was diagnosed with Ankylosing Spondylitis and my rheumatologist became my second favorite doctor, after my oncologist. Just as an aside, I cannot stress enough the importance of having a doctor who treats you as an intelligent human being whose time and health are as valuable as their own. It is demeaning and infuriating to have a doctor talk down to you and not take the time needed to understand your concerns.

Ankylosing Spondylitis (AS) is an autoimmune disease very similar to rheumatoid arthritis (RA). With any autoimmune disease, the body's immune system attacks it's own cells as if they are a foreign and threatening invader, like a bacteria or virus. The tissue, organ, or cells your body attacks will determine which autoimmune disease you manifest. Most people are familiar with RA, a crippling form of arthritis that results when your own body begins to attack the tissue in your distal (small) joints. Chronic inflammation of the joints can lead to pain, deformities, and a poor quality of life. AS operates via the same mechanism, however, the immune system attacks large joints—hips and spine—instead of small. Oh yeah, I almost forgot. For years, I had also been having recurrent "infections" in my eye. Turns out this was another autoimmune reaction called anterior UVitis where my immune system was attacking my eye and filling it with white blood cells. It is commonly associated with AS. Who knew? Certainly not any of the eye doctors I had gone to over the years. Being diagnosed with another disease just made me more committed to my anti-cancer lifestyle choices. Life went on this way for a couple of years until I was diagnosed with Crohn's disease. I will spare you the shitty (literally) details but I was told this was another autoimmune disease.

This one was causing chronic inflammation of my intestinal lining. I soldiered on in my vegetarian lifestyle and tried to convince my husband and kids that beans and rice trumped bacon and eggs on the health spectrum. Fast forward a couple of years and I had another episode of UVitis, only this time it hit with a vengeance. No amount of steroids could take away the pain and flashing lights in my eye, even after the white blood cells returned to normal. Many eye popping tests later, I was diagnosed with optic neuritis, that is, an inflamed optic nerve. Optic neuritis is a red flag for multiple sclerosis (MS). Well, I think you can guess what I am going to say next. A couple of brain scans later, and tada! I had MS too! Wait... WHAT? How was this possible? I was the best patient! I took all of my meds. I ate a healthy, vegetarian diet. I exercise almost every day. I even gave up drinking alcohol! Why was I falling apart? I thought, maybe I should try and be vegan?

As I waffled between veganism and vegetarianism (I just couldn't give up cheese and ice cream!), I stumbled upon a book called *Wheat Belly* by William Davis, MD. To say this book rocked my world is an understatement and I highly recommend you read it. Dr. Davis makes a compelling case that genetically altered wheat, even whole wheat, can cause weight gain, diabetes, heart disease, autoimmune disease, and neurological disease. This was my first introduction to gluten. I am tempted to list every book I read from this point forward, but I will spare you and include a recommended reading list at the end of this book if you are interested. Once I was pointed in the right direction, I began to learn that everything the USDA recommends in the food guide pyramid is completely backwards, and many of the nutrition principles I had adopted might have been undermining my immune system all along. For the past thirteen years, I thought I was being diagnosed with one seemingly unrelated disease after another, and I couldn't understand why! Was I that unlucky? Were my genes plagued with mutation? Now, hundreds of books, magazine articles, scientific journals, and doctor appointments later, I finally understand how and why I developed so many diseases. I really only have one problem, systemic inflammation, that has led to my many conditions. The best part is that I now understand why systemic inflammation occurs and how I can reverse it. There is so much I can do to try and control the fuel that burns the fire of my diseases. This information is not just for the sick, but for everyone interested in achieving optimal health through lifestyle choices. We are not sitting ducks! We do not have to sit by and watch our bodies deteriorate as we age. There is so much within our control and I am so excited to teach you all that I have learned.

Before you close this book wondering why you should listen to anything I have to say, let me share with you a bit about my credentials. First, and most important I believe, is that I have lived through it all. I know the fear that comes along with being diagnosed with cancer or autoimmune disease. I have lived through many surgeries, chemotherapy, several rounds of steroids, infusions, debilitating pain, and the loss of the will to live. Now, I can't wait to start my day knowing that I will attack it with my knowledge and go out into the world to share my knowledge with others. On top of that experience, I have a Bachelors of Science in Biochemistry and a Masters of Science in Biophysics and Genetics. I attended the Institute for Integrated Nutrition and am a certified Holistic Health Counselor. Everything I have learned, I have examined through the lens of a scientist. There have been many books or theories that I dismissed because I couldn't find the solid science to back it up. I am not claiming to be a doctor, but my opinion has been shaped by scientific fact. I hope you read on so I can continue to share it with you.

"Turn your wounds into wisdom."

—Oprah Winfrey

CHAPTER TWO

SO MANY DIETS, SO LITTLE TIME

Up until I was diagnosed with cancer, I had been eating the Standard American Diet, or SAD as it is appropriately called. Since the advent of the TV dinner in the early 1950s our grocery stores have become inundated with convenience foods. Instead of shopping for fresh food every few days and cooking from scratch, I was born into a generation where we could stock up on shelf stable groceries that could last for weeks, months and even years. AND the food was cheaper. AND it tasted better courtesy of food scientists whom created the perfect combination of sweet/salty/savory to ensure we would keep coming back for more. And come back we did! As a result, the incidence of heart disease, diabetes, and cancer began to skyrocket. In the early 1990s the government decided to step in and create the Food Guide Pyramid to help guide Americans to the proper way to eat. The base of the pyramid encouraged that the majority of calories come from grains, pastas, cereals and breads. Above that came fruits and vegetables. Next came meat, chicken, fish, eggs, cheese and dairy. At the tip of the pyramid, to be eaten sparingly, were fats, oils and sweets. I was out of graduate school by that time and still looking to shed my lingering freshman 15, so I dutifully adopted the high carb, low fat diet endorsed by the government. Like most of my friends and family, we believed we had upgraded our childhood diets by following the government's recommendations. Unfortunately, the disease rate continued to climb at an alarming rate.

I am pretty sure that I made a significant contribution to the success of Amazon in the dozen or so years that followed. As soon as I met my cancer surgeon, and she got wind of my endless list of questions, her first suggestion to me was to go buy a book about breast cancer. There was no way in her busy practice she was ever going to have enough time to give me all the answers I needed to move on in the cancer decision making process. However, it didn't take me long to realize that a cancer book was filled with information I didn't really want to know. I could not think of my life in terms of what statistical chance I had to be alive in 1 year, 5 years, or 10 years. So I passed those books on to my husband with instructions not to tell me anything unless it gave me information I needed to survive. I then started looking for any book, article or magazine that gave me information about cancer survival. From personal stories to scientific journals, I devoured them all. From there I concluded there was enough evidence to back up the notion that with proper lifestyle changes, mainly diet and exercise, I could stack the odds in my favor and not become another cancer statistic. With Amazon as my right hand man, I set out to become an expert in surviving cancer through diet and lifestyle changes. This quest led me down an endless road of ever growing and changing information. Lucky for me, I am an information junkie. While most people prefer to curl up in bed or go on vacation with a great novel, I was content reading about the nutritional and curative properties of superfoods. When all my friends were reading *The Kite Runner* and *Eat, Pray, Love* in their book clubs, I was home reading *Crazy, Sexy, Cancer*. This leads me not only to the reason I am writing this book, but also more specifically to why I am including this chapter in my book.

I can honestly say I have never met anyone who enjoys reading about nutrition and the etiology of disease as much as I do. But, I also have not met anyone who has not been touched, directly or indirectly, by cancer or some other lifestyle related disease like heart disease or diabetes. Plus, who doesn't want to lose a couple of pounds, have more energy, have clearer skin, and sleep better? The answers are out there people! And lucky for you, I have done all the research for you. What I want to give you in this chapter is a summary of a few of the books I have read and the diets I have tried that have been linked to improved health and disease prevention.

Chemo, surgery, read 10 books—chemo, surgery, read 10 books—within this cycle, I slowly started to make some changes. It wasn't easy, but when I finally broke up with Oscar Meyer for good, I became a vegetarian. After a couple of days, (okay, years) of whimpering when I smelled bacon, I committed myself to all things veggie. Two problems presented themselves right away: 1) what type of vegetarian was I going to be? And, 2) I had no idea how to cook! Being a vegetarian is not as straight forward as I assumed, so here's a quick overview of the different types. What all vegetarians have in common is that they avoid eating red meat. But, should I be a lacto-vegetarian, that is, a vegetarian who also eats dairy products (hello ice cream). Or, maybe an ovo-vegetarian and include eggs? Maybe I should combine the two and be a lacto-ovo-vegetarian? Then there is the question of fish. A pescatarian avoids meat but eats fish and seafood.

The pollotarian avoids red meat and fish, but eats chicken. I quickly settled on being a vegetarian who avoids all types of red meat (beef, lamb, pork, venison) as well as all types of poultry (chicken, turkey, duck). But I would allow fish, seafood, eggs and ice cream (I mean dairy). Recently, the term flexitarian has made magazine headlines and refers to individuals who try to stick to a vegetarian diet several days a week but still consume meat once in a while. Of course, what type of vegetarian you decide to be will not contribute to better health if what you end up being a junk-food-vegetarian. I have met several people on my journey who call themselves vegetarian, avoid eating meat, chicken, and/or fish, and fill their diets with french fries, fake meats, and Oreos. They are technically vegetarian but making their health worse in the process. To avoid this pitfall, I made myself a chart of what I wanted to try and include in my diet each day (i.e. vegetables, fruits, whole grains, fish, beans, flax seeds, dairy, green tea and nuts). I listed how many servings of each category I should have in a day, and after each meal, I filled out my chart. It was my first food journal of sorts and kept me focused on my small goal of making better food choices, and my larger goal of surviving cancer.

There are many incredible scientists and authors who have made it their life's work to research, accumulate data, publicize, or share their stories about the connection between poor diet and disease. This information was never offered to me by any doctor, but it is out there and not hard to find if you are willing to look. The ones I mention here are the ones that had the most significant impact on my choices, but there are many more to explore if you care to do so.

Dr. Dean Ornish, to my knowledge, was the first person to show that diet could reverse disease. This was significant because, up until his research was published, the only connection believed to exist between diet and disease was prevention. Prior to Dr. Ornish's research, there were many studies that compared what different cultures ate to the frequency of disease among different populations. Certain cultures, with certain dietary habits, had a low rate of heart disease, diabetes, and cancer. Whereas Americans, eating the SAD diet, had much higher rates of these same diseases. So, it was concluded that diet could cause or prevent lifestyle related disease. However, once disease had set in, it was there to stay...until Dean Ornish entered the picture. Dr. Dean Ornish put his sick patients on a plant heavy, very low fat, vegan diet and proved that heart disease was **reversible**! Prior to Dr. Ornish's findings, no one believed that you could make a patient better with diet and lifestyle changes alone.

This was a shocking and unexpected finding at the time. In addition to Dr. Dean Ornish, Dr. Caldwell Esselstyn has similarly proven that a plant based, oil free diet can stop the progression of heart disease and reverse its existing effects. These doctors, as well as others, have continued to prove that plant based diets can reverse heart disease, diabetes, and decrease cancer related markers like PSA.

One of my favorite authors is Kris Carr. When Kris was 31 years old, she was diagnosed with a very rare, untreatable, inoperable type of cancer. Everything about her story makes me want to stand up and yell "You go girl!" and it makes me appreciate the fact that my cancer occurred in a part of my body that doctors could cut off! Kris is the author of *Crazy, Sexy, Cancer*; *Crazy, Sexy, Cancer Tips*; *Crazy, Sexy Diet*; and *Crazy, Sexy, Kitchen*. Kris and I have had very similar journeys through disbelief, grief, fear, depression, research, discovery, reinvention, and empowerment! I was very grateful to have Kris's books to enlighten and support me along the way. Some of the things Kris and I have tried were unusual, unconventional, and made our doctor's heads spin. But I do not believe that either of us has made any mistakes. The only mistake a person can make is to sit back and become a spectator in his or her own life. I have met many people in the last decade who blindly listen to what their doctors say or, worse yet, avoid treatment out of fear. I urge you to read Kris's books. I know she will inspire you to cry, laugh, and thrive alongside her.

Enter stage left: T. Colin Campbell, PhD. T. Colin Campbell was a research scientist given the task of developing a program for a region of the Philippines whose children had an unusually high rate of liver cancer. He and his team naturally assumed that the children must be malnourished and he had to figure out a way to get more animal protein to this region of the Philippines. When Dr. Campbell and his team arrived in the Philippines with their plan, they were shocked to find out that the children with the highest rate of cancer belonged to the most affluent families. Being affluent meant they could afford higher quality food and were in fact eating a much higher percentage of animal protein compared to their peers. Dr. Campbell had grown up believing that eating animal protein made you big and strong. What he observed in the Philippines was completely opposite of that. He then made it his life's work to try and find some scientific proof of the benefits or harm associated with eating animal protein. He began with animal studies and was able to show that animals fed a diet high in casein (milk protein) developed cancer, while those fed a diet low in casein remained cancer free. Dr. Campbell then traveled to various provinces in China and discovered a direct correlation between animal protein intake and cancer incidence. As his research unfolded, Dr. Campbell became a vegan. His book, *The China Study*, is a shocking read and worth the addition to your personal library.

If you are not an avid book reader, there are many movies out there about food quality and health. One such movie that had a profound impact on the way I viewed cancer treatment was *The Gerson Miracle*. Dr. Max Gerson was a German-Jewish physician in the early 1900s. While in medical school, he suffered from severe migraine headaches. After two years of self-experimentation, he was able to eliminate his migraines completely by following a specific diet high in fruits and organic vegetables. Once Dr. Gerson introduced this diet to patients suffering from migraines, he noticed that his diet also alleviated the symptoms of skin tuberculosis. Dr. Gerson went on to cure many individuals. His most famous patients were Albert Schweitzer and his family. Dr. Gerson cured Albert Schweitzer's wife of pulmonary tuberculosis, his daughter of skin disease, and Albert of diabetes. Dr. Gerson eventually fled the persecution of Nazi Germany and settled in New York where he continued to cure many individuals of diseases considered "hopeless," including cancer. The principal theory behind Gerson therapy is to flood the body with nutrients and help it excrete toxins. This is accomplished by consuming freshly pressed, nutrient dense vegetable juices, eating organic vegetables, and taking organic coffee enemas to draw out toxins from the liver. This treatment is certainly a drastic lifestyle change, but a cancer diagnosis can make you feel desperate and willing to try just about anything! Lucky for our current generation, Dr. Gerson's daughter, Charlotte, is still continuing her father's work. She operates a clinic in Mexico and has educated and trained many holistic physicians to offer her father's therapy to their patients.

Obviously, I have greatly oversimplified the research and life experiences of Dr. Dean Ornish, Kris Carr, T. Colin Campbell, and Dr. Max Gerson. But, the conclusion they all came to by vastly different paths was that the most significant way to influence your health in a positive way is to adopt a vegan diet. And vegan I was determined to be! A vegan shuns any food that comes from an animal source including meat, poultry, fish, seafood, dairy, animal fats like lard or gelatin that come from animal bones, and eggs. Some vegans even avoid honey because it comes from bees. Outside of the food issue, many vegans take great efforts not to use commodities sourced from animals like leather or fur, as well as products like cosmetics that are created based on research involving lab animals. I entered the vegan world simply focused on its health benefits. I was largely ignorant of any of the other reasons to be vegan and, even as those reasons started to surface in my readings, I was too selfish at the time to care. I wasn't interested in being an animal activist or saving the planet. I just wanted to live long enough to raise my kids. It wasn't until I added binge watching documentaries about food to my voracious search for knowledge did that change. OMG!!! What was I thinking?! What are any of us thinking?!

It is impossible to explore the world of veganism and stay focused only on food. Factory farmed animals in America live under despicable conditions. Chickens are kept in hen houses so crowded that their beaks have to be seared off so they can't peck each other. Their feet routinely get caught and injured on the wire floors of their cages and require antibiotics to fight infection. Hormones are administered to optimize egg laying potential and to insure the maximum growth of breast muscle. Chicken breasts are allowed to grow so large that chickens are unable to support their weight and topple forward. They rarely see the sunlight and are fed cheap grain or worse instead of their natural diet of grubs and worms. Cattle are equally kept in crowded barns, knee deep in their own feces. They are fed grain instead of their natural diet of wild grass. They never see the sun. They are given hormones and artificially inseminated to keep them perpetually lactating so they can be milked as often as possible. This leads to inflamed and infected utters which are treated with potent antibiotics. To anyone reading this who has ever breastfed a baby and gotten mastitis, can you imagine being forced to breastfeed, 24/7, with a painful infection, for your entire existence? I would gladly donate my mammary glands to the cancer gods rather than endure that! After their miserable existence, they are led to slaughter. I urge you to educate yourself about factory farming. It doesn't take long. One documentary and you will be changed for life (I recommend *Vegucated* and *Forks Over Knives*). From there, every consumer choice you make that doesn't support factory farming is a step in the right direction. It is the least we can do to fight the downright criminal practices occurring in factory farms. And let's not forget the environment. Where do you think all those feces are going? Animal excrement has depleted the nutrients in our soil and created "dead zones" in our waterways where no species can survive. When a vegetable is recalled for contamination like E. coli, it is because it grew in soil soaked with animal excrement. Gross! Methane gas emitted from the backside of cattle is the number one threat to the ozone layer. Every time you make a choice to eat less meat, you are helping yourself, the animals, and the environment. Win, win, win!

Unfortunately, what my intellectual side tells me and what my food-obsessed side tells me are constantly at odds and I continue to have a very hard time committing to veganism 100%. I blame it all on ice cream! To this day, I remain a highly passionate vegan-wannabe. I share this with you because I have read many diet/health books that outline the steps you need to take in order to "lose the weight" or "get healthy." Every time I read a book that outlines a plan that makes sense to me, I commit to the plan in hopes of achieving the desired results—"Lose 7 pounds in one week!" Sounds good to me. But, I inevitably "cheat" on one or two (or ten) rules and don't achieve the holy grail promised by the book. This makes me feel like a failure! How can I cheat on a diet when I know how important it is for me to eat well so I can live longer? I have little kids I have to raise. Aren't they more important than ice cream? My point is this: NOBODY is perfect! Not even beautiful, thin Hollywood stars who live on juice cleanses. Changing the way you've eaten your entire life is hard. Choosing a different eating path, when it seems like everyone around you can eat whatever he or she wants and not get sick or gain weight, is hard. But you don't have to be perfect to be moving in the right direction. Every little choice you make can have a positive effect on your health even if you can't weigh and measure the results. Start by focusing on adding in some good things instead of what you have to give up. Most of all, be kind to yourself. Beating yourself up because you "cheated" on a diet is a waste of time and energy. There is no holy grail. Good health is a life long journey and you are your own experiment. Losing seven pounds in one week did not make me healthier, it made me hungrier! There are no mistakes. Learn from your experiments what makes you feel good, or learn from me. But keep learning!

Okay, where was I? Oh yeah, I am a vegan-wannabe! And there I have stayed for many years. As I struggled with my weight—yes, you can gain weight on a vegan diet—and continued my relentless pursuit of health and cancer information, I bid on, and won, several sessions with a holistic health counselor at my kid's school fundraiser. My health counselor, Jill, had gotten her education at the Institute for Integrative Nutrition in New York City. She was exactly what I was looking for at the time, and fed my insatiable appetite for the latest in nutrition science. Jill introduced me to nutrition concepts like macrobiotics, raw food, and Ayurveda, just to name a few. Every word out of her mouth just made me want to learn more—so much so that, I too, eventually enrolled as a student at the Institute of Integrative Nutrition (IIN). IIN is a phenomenal nutrition school in that it doesn't believe in, or teach, just one approach to nutrition, but it sets out to educate its students about EVERY nutrition concept. Woohoo! I felt like I'd hit the lottery! IIN's unique approach was founded on a belief in bioindividuality. Bioindividuality is based on the concept that one person's food can be another person's poison. In order to be an effective health counselor, you need to know about every approach to nutrition so that you are armed with enough information to help each client with his or her unique set of health challenges/beliefs/needs/concerns. Ah-ha moment! Of course! The conditions that made my body a ripe breeding ground for cancer cells was not identical to any other person diagnosed with cancer. My age, genetic predisposition, stress level, sleep patterns, eating habits, environmental exposures, were unique to me. So my approach to cancer survival, likewise, should be unique to me. I loved attending IIN. I especially loved the celebratory conga—line dance my kids, niece and nephews did every time I got a 100% on an exam. I graduated IIN armed and ready to teach others the customized nutritional approach that would help lead them to become their best, healthiest self. Unfortunately, my body had other plans for me...again.

In the years that followed, I was diagnosed with so many autoimmune diseases that I considered applying for a spot in the book of Guinness World Records. How could a dedicated vegan-wannabe still be getting so sick? To make matters worse, or better since misery loves company, my sister was diagnosed with rheumatoid arthritis. It was nice to have someone to talk to that knew what it was like to feel scared, crippled, and old before their time. Autoimmune fear and cancer fear are very different. Cancer fear hits with, "OMG, I could die tomorrow. Who is going to take care of my kids?!" Autoimmune fear hits with, "OMG, I could die after years of painful degeneration. Who's going to take care of me AND my kids?!" But my sister and I were a pretty good two-member support group and I finally had someone to call who understood my fear, pain, fatigue and relentless brain fog! However, our support for one another went beyond commiserating. Anytime each of us tried or learned something new about autoimmune disease, we shared it with the other in the hopes that it would benefit one of us. Our first joint experiment was to read and commit to trying *The Virgin Diet* by JJ Virgin. In *The Virgin Diet*, it is explained how food sensitivities or intolerances can lead to inflammation and eventually weight gain, physical symptoms, and even disease. We didn't know it at the time, but *The Virgin Diet* was just the tip of the iceberg in the explanation of how food can cause autoimmune disease. I had discovered a new focus for my crazed desire to learn everything about the diseases plaguing my life. Not long after, I came upon a book called *The Immune System Recovery Plan*. Perfect! My immune system was a mess and I wanted to recover. The book had a three-pronged approach to attacking autoimmune disease. First, figure out what foods are causing you inflammation and eliminate them. Second, cleanse your body of stored toxins. And third, take control of your stress level. Sounded simple enough, but for me, the book was totally overwhelming. I am not a hypochondriac but, I felt like I had every symptom and risk factor described in the book. I was very fortunate to discover that the author of the book, Dr. Susan Blum, had an office a little over an hour from my house so, instead of trying to figure out where to begin on my own, I decided to make an appointment at The Blum Center. It was there that I finally began to learn what was really wrong with me.

Before I could begin to take on my autoimmune disease, the Blum Center discovered I had another problem. I had an overgrowth of bad bacteria in my intestines called Candida. Our bodies are host to trillions of bacteria that play a crucial role in digestion, vitamin absorption, and toxin breakdown. But not all bacteria are "good" and the balance between good and bad can be upset by many things including (you guessed it) a bad immune system! Just Candida alone could be the cause of many of my daily symptoms like chronic fatigue and bloating. So, my first order of business became adopting an Anti-Candida Diet. Easier said than done! Candida is a form of yeast that feeds on sugar, or any carbohydrate that breaks down into sugar, once digested. The treatment, therefore, is to starve the yeast of its main fuel—sugar. In addition, peanuts and pistachios must be avoided due to their high mold content; mushrooms and anything in the fungus family can cross react with Candida; and fermented foods like vinegar, sauerkraut, and moldy cheese can provoke symptoms of Candida. And I thought giving up bacon was hard! Now I had to break up with Ben and Jerry too?! But when I lay awake at night imagining bacteria in my intestines partying like they were on spring break, giving up sugar didn't seem insurmountable. It was at this juncture that I started to realize that my diet as a vegan-wannabe was made up of mostly carbs. Well, if I had taught myself how to cook delicious beans, grains, breads, and desserts then I could now learn how to cook without them. All of my vegan and vegetarian cookbooks were loaded with carbs so I went searching for new recipes that would not feed the beast growing within.

I had heard of the paleo diet before but had never looked into it because the word paleo, in my mind, was analogous with "Unga Bunga. Me want meat!" But I also knew it was a diet that avoided grains and breads, so maybe if I ignored the meat part, I could find some delicious grain free veggie recipes. I picked up a few paleo cookbooks and was utterly shocked by what I found! Every paleo cookbook began with an intro written by an author who had suffered from autoimmune disease and found their way back to health through the paleo diet. Come again? What on earth did paleo have to do with autoimmune disease? I scoured the internet and Amazon for more info and read every paleo book I could get my hands on. Individuals who follow the paleo diet eat in a way that is consistent with what was available to our ancestors prior to agriculture. Until about 10,000 years ago, humans ate only what they could hunt or forage for. That is, meat, fish, fruits, vegetables, nuts and seeds. Once we developed the ability to stay in one place and grow food, our diets drastically changed. Grains and dairy became a significant source of calories and alleviated the stress of not knowing where or when the next meal was going to come from. This change was potentially life saving at the time, but laid the groundwork for deterioration in our health that we wouldn't fully realize for thousands of years. To make matters worse, the past 100 years have managed to change our food supply into something unrecognizable to our earlier ancestors. First, we introduced factory farming, canning, and pesticides, followed by refined sugar and flour. This opened the floodgates and in poured fast food, TV dinners, and the ability to process and package everything you could imagine. To make sure the nails were securely positioned to hold our coffins shut, we decided to start giving our animals hormones and antibiotics and genetically engineering our crops.

It doesn't take a science degree to see that something is seriously wrong with our food system now. My favorite Paleo book, however, was written by a scientist. *The Paleo Approach: Reverse Autoimmune Disease and Heal Your Body* by Sarah Ballantyne is a mind scrambling collection of information that dissects every aspect of how post agriculture foods have attacked our bodies. Sarah has a PhD in medical biophysics so, at last, someone was talking my language. *The Paleo Approach* is a biochemistry textbook from start to finish. Finally, I wasn't being told to eat a certain way to combat disease without a scientific explanation. Now I had hardcore biochemistry to back up why I had inflammation running amok in my body, how it caused autoimmune disease, and what I had to change in order to get well again. And by the way, I kicked those Candida bugs out of the party in no time flat!

"I like living. I have sometimes been wildly, despairingly, acutely miserable, racked with sorrow, but through it all I still know quite certainly that just to be alive is a grand thing."

—Agatha Christie

CHAPTER THREE
LEAKY WHAT?

Despite spending a decade reading about the connection between food and illness, I still had a lot to learn. My real answers finally came in the form of something called Leaky Gut Syndrome. Leaky what? Why haven't I come across this concept before? I had been going to gastroenterologists for years, had tubes and cameras exploring my innards more times than I wish to remember, but never, EVER was the term leaky gut even hinted at. I was stunned. I was pissed off! But most of all, I was so thankful that I finally had answers—real scientific answers that applied directly to me. And guess what, they probably apply to you or someone you know too!

I now know that I have Leaky Gut Syndrome and that my leaky gut is the underlying reason why I developed autoimmune disease. I am not saying that it's why I developed ankylosing spondylitis (AS) or, that it's why I developed Crohn's disease. I am saying it's why I developed every single one of my autoimmune diseases, and possibly contributed to why I developed cancer as well. In fact, I learned that leaky gut is the reason why ALL autoimmune diseases occur. Let me say that again. If you have an autoimmune disease of any kind, you definitely have a leaky gut. Yes, you read that correctly. If you have autoimmune thyroid disease, lupus, rheumatoid arthritis, psoriatic arthritis, multiple sclerosis, vitiligo, celiac disease, scleroderma, sarcoidosis, peripheral neuropathy, Crohn's disease—ANY autoimmune disease—you also have Leaky Gut Syndrome. Leaky gut is what allows autoimmune disease to develop.

We all have a general knowledge of our digestive system. We eat food, begin digesting it in our mouths when we chew, swallow it down into our stomach where acids digest it further, and then it is sent into our intestines. In our small intestine, we digest further and absorb vital nutrients important for brain function, muscle building, cell repair, bone strength, hormone balance, organ function, and fat storage. The process is completed in our large intestines and what remains is excreted as waste. Our intestines are semi-permeable so that we absorb the proper nutrients from our food. That is, they have a sophisticated barrier system that allows nutrients out into our blood and lymph system while keeping undigested food, bacteria, and toxins in. When this barrier system is compromised, the tight junctions holding the cells together open up and allow foreign substances to pass through the intestinal lining and "leak" out of our intestines. The end result is Leaky Gut Syndrome.

Our immune system is very efficient at attacking foreign invaders and protecting and healing us from bacterial and viral infections. Unfortunately, substances that leak out of our intestines and into our bodies are viewed by our immune system as just as foreign as any infection because they aren't supposed to be there. The army that makes up our immune system marches in our defense, attacks the enemy invader, and leaves inflammation in its wake. Normally, this process is vital to our survival, however, once leaky gut is present, our immune system remains in battle mode meal after meal, and inflammation becomes chronic. Chronic inflammation is associated with virtually every disease including heart disease, diabetes, and cancer but does not directly cause autoimmune disease. Autoimmune disease develops because of something called molecular mimicry.

When our immune system responds to a foreign invader, it creates antibodies specific to the surface structure of each invader. Like a lock and key, each antibody fits perfectly around the invader and proceeds to destroy it. Once a specific antibody is made, a future infection by the same invader is dealt with much faster because the body recognizes it from previous infections and has the specific antibody ready and waiting. When you have Leaky Gut Syndrome, antibodies are repeatedly attacking foreign proteins, bacteria, and toxins with each meal. Molecular mimicry occurs when two molecules are so similar in shape that the antibody released to attack recognizes both as the same and fits both equally. Both molecules mimic each other enough that our immune system can't tell them apart. Autoimmune disease develops because many of the substances present in our intestines look identical to our immune system as our own cells. For example, if you eat a bagel and some undigested proteins leak out of your intestines into your blood, and those particles look exactly the same on the surface as cells in your brain, your immune system, while trying to fight what's leaking out of your intestines, will also start to attack similar looking cells in your brain. If leaky gut persists and, like most people, you continue to eat similar foods every day, these brain cells will become damaged over time. The result of this damage could cause multiple sclerosis. This scenario applies to every autoimmune disease. If your body is attacking something that mimics your thyroid cells, you could develop Hashimoto's thyroiditis or Grave's disease. If your body is attacking something that mimics cells in your joints, you could develop rheumatoid arthritis, and so on. This mechanism explains why one problem, a leaky gut, can cause EVERY autoimmune disease and why, if an autoimmune disease exists, we can assume that a leaky gut existed first.

The absolute best part of what I just told you is that leaky gut is not a permanent condition. You can heal your gut and, for many people, this can lead to reversal of their autoimmune disease! Imagine that. Millions of people are suffering from autoimmune disease and it's potentially reversible. Let's take a look at what causes leaky gut in the first place and what we can do about it. Our bodies produce a protein called zonulin (sounds like a species on Star Trek) that controls the tight junctions lining our intestinal wall. Remember, these junctions allow important nutrients out while keeping the rest inside our intestines. Anything that disrupts the function of zonulin has the ability to disrupt, or loosen, those tight junctions, allowing foreign particles to leak out of our intestines. In addition, anything that has the potential to trigger a response from our immune system once it has leaked out of our gut can eventually lead to autoimmune disease. The number one substance that disrupts zonulin and also stimulates the immune system is... drumroll, please...gluten.

I have no doubt that you have heard the term gluten by now. Suddenly, grocery stores are carrying hundreds of gluten-free cookies, breads, pasta. Even some restaurants are offering a gluten-free menu. Seems like the next Hollywood fad diet has arrived in the form of gluten. For many people, that's all it is, a fad diet. But there is more to going gluten-free than just seeing if it's another possible path to losing weight. Gluten is a combination of proteins that are present in all forms of wheat, rye, barley, kamut, spelt, and triticale. Any food made with these grains, whether they are processed or whole, contain gluten. When gluten is eaten, it has the ability to irritate the lining of the intestinal wall, stimulate an overproduction of zonulin, loosen the tight junctions regulating what is held in the intestines, leak out of the intestines, and trigger an immune response that can lead to mild, moderate, or severe symptoms. Individuals who have a severe reaction to gluten, or a gluten allergy, develop Celiac disease which permanently damages the lining of the intestinal wall. The only treatment for Celiac disease is 100% removal of all gluten-containing grains from the diet. Individuals who have a more mild response to gluten, a sensitivity or intolerance, may or may not be aware of symptoms or the silent inflammation brewing in their bodies until the onset of an autoimmune disease. A gluten sensitivity or intolerance can go undiagnosed for a lifetime because inflammation is silent, or symptoms are occurring in a part of the body that has no logical connection whatsoever with your intestines. For example, gluten intolerance has been linked to acne, ADHD, asthma, brain fog, congestion, depression, achy joints, fatigue, headaches, inability to lose weight, moodiness, skin rashes... and the list goes on and on. There are so many symptoms that we just learn to accept as part of aging, or from lack of sleep, or as part of "just the way we are." What a relief it would be if we could feel better just by eliminating gluten from our diet. Not to mention the amazing ability to potentially prevent or reverse autoimmune disease!

I wish that was all there is to it. Never eat gluten again and never be sick again. Of course, it's not that simple. But don't get discouraged! The more information you have, the more tools you have to make yourself well. There happen to be many foods that contribute to the formation of leaky gut and are capable of stimulating the immune system. These include all grains, legumes (beans), nuts and seeds.

What all these foods have in common is that they all play a role in sprouting the next generation of plant, grass or tree. When a grain or seed falls to the ground, they sprout and grow into another plant. Simple, right? Well, just like humans protect their young at all costs, plants have developed a protective mechanism to assure the highest likelihood of reproduction. All grains, legumes, nuts and seeds have either a toxic protein coating or an indigestible property to them. This helps to deter animals from eating them and, if they do get eaten, they remain undigested. That way, when the animal poops, the intact seed lands back on the ground and is still able to sprout into a new plant. Nature is amazing. Unfortunately, humans decided not too long ago that it would be a good idea to grow grains and beans for food. Their mildly toxic and indigestible properties affect us by contributing to leaky gut and stimulating our immune system. In the animal kingdom, the mildly toxic, reproductive "seed" that we eat is called eggs. Eggs can potentially trigger our immune system as well. And just to make the list complete, dairy products also cause increased intestinal permeability as well as vegetables belonging to the nightshade family, i.e., tomatoes, potatoes, peppers and eggplant. (If you are a science geek like me, the biochemical mechanism behind every trigger of intestinal permeability is laid out in detail in *The Paleo Approach* by Sarah Ballantyne.)

So, what's a food obsessed vegan-wannabe supposed to eat now? No gluten, grains, beans, nuts, seeds, dairy, nightshade veggies or eggs? But that's what most of my diet is made of. I have been living on rice and beans for a dozen years now, following dutifully my twelve servings of "healthy whole grains" just like the government food guide pyramid recommends! If gluten and grains cause leaky gut, and leaky gut causes autoimmune disease, no wonder I am the poster child for autoimmune disease. I was totally overwhelmed. The recommended diet for someone with autoimmune disease is meat, chicken, fish, fruits and vegetables. But I can't eat meat or chicken— uugh! Yet, I knew I had no choice. And with all the biochemistry backing it up, I knew this was the answer I had been looking for. The first beneficiary of my new found knowledge was my sister. Unlike me, who won't do anything without scientific facts to back it up, when I told my sister I was convinced I'd found an answer that might help us to get better, she replied, "I don't want to know why and I don't have time to read another book, so just tell me what to do." I copied a "what to eat/what not to eat" page from Sarah Ballantyne's book and mailed it to her. A few months later I was still trying to convince myself to try eating a bite of steak. However, my sister was feeling great, had lost 20 pounds, and was talking to her rheumatologist about weaning off of her RA medications. Holy smokes, it worked! I'd better get my act in gear. I went gluten, grain, bean and dairy free. Once in a while I considered taking a bite of the steak I had grilled for my boys. Okay, baby steps. Here's where things get really exciting. For as long as I can remember, my C-reactive protein has been measuring between 45 and 65. C-reactive protein is an indirect measurement of inflammation in your body. The normal range is between 0 and 4. Each time I got my results it depressed me. I couldn't believe that with all the lifestyle changes I had made since my cancer diagnosis, my C-reactive protein was still sky high. Once, during a prolonged Crohn's attack, my C-reactive protein was 400. 400! My lab report said I was at high risk for a "sudden cardiac event." Really? Now I'm going to croak from a heart attack? Anyway, after going gluten, grain, bean and dairy free for a few months, my C-reactive protein was 2.36! Words cannot express the joy, relief, and hope I experienced for the first time in a dozen years. I danced. I cried. And I vowed never to touch gluten again.

What does all this mean for you? If you have an autoimmune disease, ANY autoimmune disease, you absolutely must take steps to heal your leaky gut. I am sharing my personal experience in this book because I want you to know there are answers out there and to give you hope that you can feel better than you do right now. But, I realize I am only offering the tip of the iceberg here. If you feel like you need someone to guide you through the steps necessary to fight your autoimmune disease, please go to www.functionalmedicine.org and find a qualified doctor in you area. In America we practice "western medicine." Our doctors are trained in medical school how to diagnose disease and treat the symptoms with medication and surgery. Technology has advanced to such a degree that it is possible to live for a long time with acute or chronic illness. Just like any specialist, doctors that practice functional medicine have attended regular medical school and then have trained further to become experts in functional medicine. Instead of treating symptoms with drugs and surgery, an MD trained in functional medicine strives to uncover what went wrong in the body in the first place that eventually led to the symptom or disease. For example, a gastroenterologist typically treats Crohn's disease with various medications to manage the symptoms. When medication isn't enough, surgery is sometimes performed to remove the inflamed portion of the intestines. A functional medicine doctor would ask what caused the Crohn's disease to develop and try to treat that instead. Likewise, cancer is treated with radiation, chemotherapy and surgery. A functional medicine doctor would ask what caused the cancer to develop in the first place. I don't know about you but, this approach makes a lot of sense to me and I believe will be the direction medicine moves in the future. At least, I hope so. I am not advocating for you to walk away from your current doctor. I still believe there is a time and place for medication, chemotherapy and surgery. Just make sure you explore every option to wellness.

Now, what about if you don't have autoimmune disease? I believe that the majority of Americans are walking around with some symptom that gets in the way of feeling great every day. Whether it's brain fog, chronic congestion, migraine headaches, skin rashes, depression, a bloated belly, fatigue, diarrhea, constipation, insomnia, ADHD, achy joints, you name it, everybody has something. And let's face it, the Standard American Diet is the perfect setup for a leaky gut, even if you are trying to eat well by following the food guide pyramid. A breakfast made of an egg white omelet, lunch of a lean turkey sandwich with no mayo and hold the fries, mid-afternoon snack of greek yogurt, and pasta with vegetables for dinner creates a perfect storm for leaky gut even though it sounds like the ideal healthy diet day according to the USDA. Before leaky gut leads to full blown autoimmune disease, food sensitivities or intolerances can cause a myriad of symptoms that you have probably just learned to live with. If you are sick and tired of feeling sick or tired, here's what you need to do. You need to do an elimination diet. In an elimination diet, you take out all the foods that most commonly lead to food sensitivities for three weeks. Then, one at a time, you reintroduce each food for a few days to see if you develop any symptoms. It takes only a couple of months to complete an elimination diet and it has the potential to erase symptoms that you may have been suffering from for years! The foods commonly avoided in an elimination diet are gluten, eggs, soy, corn, dairy, peanuts, sugar and artificial sweeteners. Believe me, I know how hard it is to give up food that you love. Eating is my happy place so I understand! But I promise you it will be totally worth it. There are many books out there that guide you through the process of an elimination diet, but my favorite is *The Virgin Diet* by JJ Virgin. Holistic health counselors and functional medical doctors are well qualified to guide you through the process as well. And if you live in northern New Jersey, I can help you myself! One last thing. When you look back on the triggers for leaky gut, and the foods that cause sensitivities, doesn't it remind you of the foods that are avoided in the paleo diet? No wonder paleo people feel so good!

"Pain is inevitable. Suffering is optional."

—Haruki-Murakami

.

CHAPTER FOUR
THE WHITE DEVIL

No, I'm not talking about Jim Carey in *Ace Ventura, Pet Detective* where Ace is trying to find the sacred bat and the natives call him the White Devil. I am talking about the White Devil that taunts me day and night. The White Devil that seduces me into thinking I can have him and my health too. The White Devil that induces greed and gluttony and sloth. The White Devil that produces glee one minute, only to drop me down into despair and self-loathing the next. The White Devil, for me, is sugar.

I know sugar is bad for me. I know it can make me fat. And I know it makes me act irrationally (like hiding in the closet and polishing off a box of Girl Scout cookies when no one is looking). I swear that I look forward to Halloween more than my kids do because they arrive with bags full of candy and I don't even have to walk around and collect it myself. One of the best perks of parenting for sure! I have sworn off sugar dozens of times. I have even given it up for Lent every year for as long as I can remember. And yet, no matter how hard I try, I just can't seem to break free of my addiction. Even after saying goodbye to pizza, bagels, linguini and all things gluten, sugar still has a hold on me.

Let's take a look at how sugar works in the body and why it has the ability to turn a rational, intelligent person into a crazy, sugar seeking zombie (or maybe that's just me?) Glucose is the simple sugar that all carbohydrates are broken down into and it is the primary fuel for your brain and your muscles. In short, we can't live without it. But if we look back in history, for millions of years, the sugar we consumed consisted largely of complex carbs, like vegetables and seasonal, low sugar fruits like berries. Our DNA is programmed to allow us to process a small amount of sugar and keep our brains and muscles at peek performance. However, while our DNA has remained largely unchanged from our ancient selves, our diet has become inundated with simple carbs and sugar. When we eat carbs, or sugar directly, it is converted into glucose. Our pancreas then releases a hormone called insulin. It is insulin's job to take sugar from our blood and deliver it to our brain and other parts of our body for fuel. Some additional sugar is converted into a different form called glycogen and stored in our liver and muscles for future use. There is limited storage space in our liver and muscles for glycogen. The excess glucose is stored in our body in the form of fat. We have an unlimited ability to store excess glucose as fat. Really?! Our blood glucose levels must stay in a relatively narrow range and it is insulin that maintains this important balance. When your blood sugar levels begin to drop, a hormone called glucagon signals the release of glycogen from your liver or muscles to bring blood sugar levels back into the normal range. Glucagon is typically released during exercise, when you are hungry, or when you have a high protein, low carb meal. This delicate balance of sugar storage and release worked perfectly for millions of years. Our diets of simple carbs (sugar), washed down with soda, juice or alcohol (sugar), and capped off with dessert (sugar), has pushed this balance beyond its capacity and created a big mess.

Sugar messes with your pancreas. By eating the Standard American Diet, high in carbs and sugar, we call on our pancreas to release insulin repeatedly everyday. This is a heavy burden for our pancreas as it was not designed to have to work that hard. Eventually, our pancreas gets so overworked and fatigued that it starts losing its ability to sense changes in blood sugar levels. This is called insulin resistance. If the pancreas continues to be overworked, day after day, week after week, meal after meal, it will eventually give out and stop producing insulin all together. But our blood sugar levels still need to be kept in that perfect range, which is why someone would need to take insulin injections. This condition is called type 2 diabetes. Type 2 diabetes used to be an adult onset disease. However, our diets have become so poor in the last decade that children as young as age 5 are being diagnosed as diabetic. (Type 1 diabetes refers to a genetic condition in which the pancreas is unable to produce insulin.)

Sugar messes with your hormones. Our high carb, high sugar diets call on our pancreas repeatedly to lower our blood sugar levels. This creates an ongoing rollercoaster ride of sugar highs and resulting lows. This makes me elated when I'm binge eating gluten free muffins, and then wishing I had the ability to take a nap shortly thereafter. This rollercoaster is perceived by our bodies as a metabolic stress, and as a result, we produce a hormone called cortisol. Cortisol is the stress hormone that gives us an extra burst of energy in an emergency situation. This response was designed to aid us during times of intense, temporary stress like an encounter with a bear in the woods. Cortisol helps to regulate other bodily functions, like digestion, so we can focus on the urgent task at hand—survival. For millions of years, cortisol provided us with a much needed advantage when being chased by a wild animal or enemy tribe. This stress was intense, but short lived. Sugar consumption on the other hand, creates a state of chronic, low level stress in our bodies that is ongoing. An intense burst of cortisol is what our DNA is coded to handle. Steady levels of cortisol instead send signals to our body to store fat and decrease production of other hormones like thyroid and sex hormones. So, ladies, if you crave Ben and Jerry's more than your husband, it's not your fault! To add insult to injury, chronically elevated cortisol levels cause leaky gut. Two other hormones, called leptin and ghrelin are responsible for signaling your brain when you are full (leptin) and when you are hungry (ghrelin). When sugar consumption remains high you develop leptin and/or ghrelin resistance which prompts you to keep eating even when you are full. (I prefer to call ghrelin, gremlin, since the hunger gremlins are always chasing me.) This state of hormone deregulation is meant to be temporary and life saving, not constant and blubber creating.

Sugar messes with your gut. Sugar feeds the bad kind of yeast that inhabit your intestines. Remember the Candida diet I had to do that eliminated all forms of sugar and simple carbs? Sugar also feeds other nasty bacteria in your intestines and sets you up for an unfavorable ratio of bad bacteria to good bacteria. This imbalance can cause dysbiosis or a condition called SIBO (small intestinal bacterial overgrowth). These conditions can lead to a myriad of symptoms ranging from gas and bloating to nutrient deficiencies. Good bacteria are essential for proper digestion and nutrient absorption. A functional medicine doctor can test your bacterial flora and determine what you need to do to regain a healthy balance.

Sugar messes with your brain. Sugar has the ability to produce the same addictive effect on the brain as illegal street drugs. In other words, when you eat sugar, you crave more sugar. Sugar also affects chemicals in your brain called serotonin and dopamine. Serotonin is a "feel good" chemical that helps you to sleep well, have fewer headaches, and maintain a positive attitude. Dopamine is a neurotransmitter responsible for feelings of pleasure and excitement. This is why they call it a "sugar high." When sugar decreases, your brain makes you crave more sugar so that you can feel that "high" again. Our DNA was programmed to make us seek out sweet flavors because sweetness was traditionally associated with nutrient density. For example, eating berries would include a pleasing sweet flavor and a strong nutritional punch, which provided copious vitamins and minerals needed for survival. But sweet berries were hard to come by and seasonal millions of years ago. Now, however, not only can we buy berries year round, but sugar is readily available to us in a variety of cheap and easily accessible forms. Since I don't know many people who go on a berry binge, I think it's safe to say that our steady consumption of sugar comes primarily from sources void of any nutrients, leaving our brains still searching for the anticipated nutrition it was expecting from sweet flavor. The end result... more cravings.

Sugar messes with your immune system. If we eat high calorie, low nutrient meals when our bodies are programmed to expect calories and nutrients to come together, our systems are thrown into a state of metabolic stress. This stress causes inflammation. Likewise, riding the sugar high/low rollercoaster causes stress, which causes inflammation. Chronically increased insulin causes stress, which causes inflammation. You get the picture. Sugar = stress = inflammation. Inflammation undermines our immune system which directly leads to all types of disease including heart disease, autoimmune disease, diabetes, and even cancer.

A discussion on sugar would not be complete without

a word about artificial sweeteners. Since our bodies are programmed to associate sweetness with calories and nutrients, artificial sweeteners somehow try to trick us by providing sweetness without calories OR nutrients. Unfortunately, our brains rebel by making us crave more calories. This is why you may have heard about recent reports that say drinking diet soda can actually make you gain weight. Although your soda has no calories, you may end up eating more just to satisfy the mixed messages you are sending your brain. In addition, artificial sweeteners have been linked to migraines, dizziness, seizures, nausea, diarrhea, fatigue, mood swings, vision problems, irregular heart rate, joint pain, loss of memory, insomnia, and skin rashes. I don't know about you but artificial sweeteners sound like the White Devil's evil twin.

Before I leave the topic of sugar, I'd like to mention the glycemic index. The glycemic index was developed as a tool to measure how quickly sugars from food are released into the bloodstream. Sounds very useful, especially for someone with diabetes, generalized inflammation, or even someone just wanting to lose a few pounds. Unfortunately, the glycemic index looked at all food on an equal playing ground, regardless of portion size. And you and I know it's a lot easier to overeat a warm basket of bread than a bowl of carrots. To compensate for this flaw, the glycemic load was created, which is a more accurate look at how a particular food will affect blood sugar based on a realistic portion size. Take watermelon for example. Its glycemic index is high, but when portion size is added to the equation, the glycemic load is low. The glycemic load can be helpful for someone who really needs a number to guide his or her choices. But if you avoid sugar and food made from grains that turn quickly into sugar when digested, I don't think you need to obsess over the glycemic index, or load, of everything you put in your mouth. Wait a minute, no sugar or grains? That sounds a lot like the paleo diet, again!

I am not the kind of person who can take a taste of a dessert and leave the rest on the plate. I hate those people! Once the White Devil passes my lips, I commence the feeding frenzy until not a morsel remains. I accept that the White Devil will continue to haunt me for the rest of my life. And, with its ability to sabotage my pancreas, hormones, brain, gut, and immune system, I understand that I will never be truly healthy until I exorcise it from my soul. Easier said than done, I know. But I am committed to fight the evil hold it has on me every hour, every day, every year, for as long as it takes. I hope that you will join me in my crusade.

"There are only two ways to live your life. One is as though nothing is a miracle. The other is as though everything is a miracle."

—Albert Einstein

CHAPTER FIVE

DEM BONES

For all the hardcore vegans out there reading this book, I want to apologize in advance for this chapter about—Eeww!—animal bones. About six months into my education about all things paleo, I still wasn't eating any meat. But after seeing the incredible results my sister was having on the paleo diet, I knew I had to make a bigger effort to embrace this new lifestyle. I bought paleo cookbooks, shopped for 100% grass fed beef, cooked the recipes from scratch, and then served it to everyone in the family...except myself. Something about looking at the meat uncooked, (which I would only touch with latex gloves on) was enough for me to talk myself out of my mission to go paleo. Maybe I should just order meat in a restaurant so I don't have to look at it, or touch it, before it is cooked? But then, I knew, it wouldn't be of the grass-fed, free-range, wild, quality I was looking for. As my vegan and paleo minions battled it out in my brain, I received a very timely email from The Natural Gourmet Institute in New York City. They were offering a class to lay people, that is, people not enrolled in their culinary degree program called "A Four Day Paleo Intensive Cooking Class." Great! Maybe if I were taught by real chefs how to cook paleo, and everything tasted as if a professional chef had cooked it, I would have an easier time making the transition. Right then and there, before I had time to worry about how I was going to get my kids to and from school and activities, I signed up to spend four days in New York, cooking—yikes—meat!

DAY 1—Slow Cooking Bone Broths & Fermentation

I was ecstatic to find out that the instructor was Myra Kornfeld. Myra is a professional chef and author of the fabulous vegan cookbook The Voluptuous Vegan. A vegan cookbook writer teaching a paleo cooking class? Maybe I'm not the only one with paleo-vegan thoughts pulling me in different directions? The first thing we did on day one was introduce ourselves. I was most certainly out of my league. Most of the other "students" were professional chefs or health coaches looking to boost their careers with a broader range of knowledge. I was trying to learn how to look at a piece of raw meat without gagging. I had promised myself that I was going to cook, touch, and taste everything put in front of me. So it began. We roasted and simmered bones, ribs, knuckles, backs, wings, necks, feet, and whole carcasses—ugh! When Myra mentioned the option to clip the nails of the chicken feet before boiling, I almost quit the class right then and there. After the dismembered animals were quietly stewing away, we moved on to fermentation. First, we strained the liquid whey out of yogurt to use as the fermentation agent and then proceeded to make fermented drinks, salsa and chutney. Since fermentation and bone broth take several days to create, there was no tasting to be done on day one. Phew!

DAY 2—Braising, Preparing Nuts & Grains, Grinding Flours

Although I hadn't fallen in love with paleo cooking yet, I was quickly becoming a fan of Myra Kornfeld. She had an incredible wealth of knowledge and was genuinely interested and engaged in helping all of us learn. She taught us all about nuts, seeds, grains, and legumes with a focus on their anti-nutrient and indigestible properties. She reinforced what I had learned about the causes of leaky gut and why a paleo diet avoids grains and beans. Then she taught us that by soaking, sprouting, fermenting, and cooking them that we could reduce the amount of potentially harmful qualities. I was very excited to hear that perhaps, after I heal my leaky gut, I might be able to reintroduce grains and beans back into my diet by implementing the proper soaking techniques. After our mini seminar, we began to cook, and cook, and cook. We used our bone broths from day one to make butternut squash soup, beet borsht, French onion soup, and cioppino. We braised lamb necks, short ribs, lamb shanks, fish, and chicken. Lastly, we made a simple green salad (thank God). True to the promise I had made myself when I put my credit card number in the computer upon registration, I tasted everything! All the soups were AMAZING! I never would have known that the butternut squash soup had a backbone. The rest, well, I had a ways to go. But I loved the salad!

DAY 3—Homemade Nut Butters, Organ Meats

The first part of the class had me crafting elaborate excuses why I was too ill to continue and deserved a full refund. We made duck confit, liver paté, chicken liver with caramelized onions, and roasted bone marrow. And yes, I tasted everything! But the second half of the class—jackpot! We made gluten free waffles, crepes, crackers, porridge, sourdough bread, scrambled eggs, and nut butters with our pre-soaked nuts from day two, I gobbled up everything sans gluten and was in my happy place once again.

DAY 4—Grain—Free Baking, Long Fermentation

I didn't think we could top day three but, on day four, we baked paleo pancakes, coconut flour bread, cauliflower muffins, flourless carrot-almond muffins, flax-nut muffins, date-nut loaf, coconut breakfast muffins, raw fudge, chia seed pudding, and fresh nut milk. Everything was gluten free, grain free, and YUMMY! To conclude our four-day smorgasbord, we each made our own jar of kraut to ferment on our countertops at home and we learned how to make kombucha. Now, I have been witnessing kombucha appear on the shelves of Whole Foods for some time, had heard it was good for you, but had no clue as to what it actually was. According to Myra, kombucha has the ability to break down and digest food, decrease toxicity, inhibit growth of bad microorganisms, relieve joint pain, act as an anti-spasmodic, and bring the body into balance so it can heal itself. Wow! I've got to try that! Kombucha is a drink that is fermented by a symbiotic colony of bacteria called a scoby. A scoby looks like a giant, extremely slimy, Portobello mushroom. To make kombucha, tea bags and sugar are added to water and the scoby is placed on top to ferment. This large jar is covered with a cloth that allows air in for the scoby to breathe. Really? Isn't there a less disgusting way to get all those fabulous health benefits? And then, faster than you can say "kombucha, kimchi, kvass," my whirlwind cooking experience ended and I found myself running for the train—kraut in one hand and a scoby in the other.

I was lucky to have had a long train ride home every day to process all that I had learned and contemplate whether or not I was going to incorporate my new paleo knowledge and skills into my lifestyle. I was eager to share what I had learned with my family and over the next few months I made fruit kvass, date nut loaf, French onion soup, braised chicken, several batches of bone broth, and, yes, I even made liver paté. The scoby, on the other hand, met its doom. It's been an interesting culinary adventure since the class as my vegan conscience battled my new paleo knowledge. In the end, I have realized that I am not destined to become a meat eater again. My desire to be a vegan has planted itself deep within all that I am. But medically, I still understand my need to avoid gluten, grains, beans, and dairy. And a vegan diet without those staples, is, well...sparse. So I have settled in on a compromise, one that hopefully balances my passion for veganism with my medical needs.

My big compromise, in two words, is...bone broth. I had read about slow cooked bone broth in all the paleo books but the cooking class really took my understanding to another level. If we look back in time to the thousands of generations that came before us, our ancestors made use of every part of the animal by preparing broth or stock from its bones. It is only recently that we started buying individual filets of beef or boneless chicken breasts. Just like many changes that have occurred in our modern food supply, the use of homemade broths from animal bones has virtually disappeared from American cooking. I can remember my mother, who grew up in South America, breaking chicken bones to suck out the marrow. I thought that was gross when I was a child, still do, but it never occurred to me that it might be nutritious. I doubt my mom thought of it as nutritious either. It simply was the way she was raised; not to waste any part of the animal. I am sure many of you can recall a grandmother who boiled bones too. Most cultures have held the traditional belief that bone broths provide protection from many health problems including infections, fatigue, arthritis, thyroid imbalance, mood disorders, anemia and more.

As it turns out, properly prepared bone broth made from grass-fed, free-range, or wild animals is loaded with nutrients. Boiling bones for several hours extracts minerals, collagen, cartilage, marrow, and gelatin from the bones. Adding acidity, like vinegar, to the cooking water helps to pull calcium, magnesium, potassium, and amino acids into the broth. When the broth is done cooking and allowed to cool, it has a jelly like consistency from all the gelatin. Gelatin can help heal and protect the lining of the digestive tract (goodbye leaky gut!) When your digestive tract is healthy you absorb more nutrients from your food, including protein. So adding bone broth to a "meatless" diet allows you to fully utilize the protein that you do consume. The calcium and minerals in bone broth can also help to build up your bones. No milk mustache required. Bone broth helps fight inflammation, a prerequisite to most disease and definitely a raging fire in mine. Glucosamine is a popular supplement synthetically made to help reduce joint pain but it occurs naturally in bone broth. Not to mention that the collagen and gelatin help to strengthen hair and nails. You might ask how I can call myself a vegan-wannabe and justify the use of animal bones. It was a decision born out of necessity, NOT desire, and is still not an easy one for me. But I realize I need to do everything in my power to heal my gut or I am going to go down in a ball of inflammation.

At NGI, I learned that organ meat, especially liver, is insanely nutrient dense. Liver provides more nutrients, gram for gram, than any other food. It is an excellent source of high quality protein, vitamin A, all the B vitamins (including B12 which strict vegans need to take in supplement form), folic acid (important before conception and in early pregnancy to prevent neural tube defects), iron, trace elements like copper, CoQ10 (important for cardiovascular function), and purines (precursors to DNA and RNA). Liver, in fact, is the most potent natural multivitamin around. You would think, with that resume, I'd be eating liver every day! But no, I still can't wrap my head, or hands, or teeth, around it.

Fermented foods, on the other hand, I have become a huge fan of—minus the scoby. Fermentation is another food technique that's been around for thousands of generations. Originally used as a way to preserve food, fermentation has remained a staple because of its tremendous health benefits. Even the Standard American Diet contains remnants of traditionally fermented foods like yogurt, sauerkraut, and pickles. Fermented foods provide enzymes that aid in digestion. They have a higher vitamin level than their unfermented version. They produce natural antibiotics and anti-carcinogens (my personal favorite). They help maintain regular blood pressure and heart rate, break fats down in the liver, and balance acidity in the body. They also boost the immune system by promoting the growth of healthy bacteria in the intestines. No down side as far as I can see, unless you consider eating live bacteria non-vegan? I have no idea.

I have come a long way since the Standard American Diet of my upbringing. From vegetarian to vegan-wannabe to paleo-have-to-be. Intellectually, morally, and environmentally, I remain in the vegan camp. But I have begun to boil bones on a regular basis, I eat fish occasionally for the Omega 3, and I have eggs once in a blue moon. And because my daughter works in an ice cream parlor, and sometimes I like to visit her, order a scoop, and give her a nice fat tip, I still eat ice cream on occasion. (Okay, I am just using my daughter as an excuse!) Does all of this make me a flexitarian now? Maybe so. But I prefer to call it Paleo-Vegan Yum!

"*Never doubt that a small group of thoughtful, committed, citizens can change the world. Indeed, it is the only thing that ever has.*"

—Margaret Mead

CHAPTER SIX
WAPF

WAPF stands for the Weston A. Price Foundation. I first learned about Weston Price when I attended the Institute for Integrative Nutrition. I relearned about him when I attended cooking classes at the Natural Gourmet Institute in New York City. And he has been referenced in dozens of the books and articles I have read pertaining to the connection between food and health. Weston Price was a dentist who, nearly 100 years ago, set out to find an answer as to why he was seeing a steady increase in dental caries (cavities), oral and facial bone deformities, and occlusion (crowding) of teeth. His research was so far reaching, and his findings so astounding, that I felt compelled to summarize them here. If you are fascinated by his findings, as I was, and would like more than just a quick summary, please read his book *Nutrition and Physical Degeneration.*

Dr. Price became more and more concerned about the increase in dental problems among his patients. He also held the belief that the health status of your mouth directly correlates to the health of the rest of your body. But instead of spending his time studying his ill patients, he had a novel approach to the problem. He decided to travel to remote tribes and villages around the world and study cultures that were free from the dental abnormalities he was seeing in his practice. Why were they free of cavities, crowding, and deformities? Why did they seem to be blessed with robust health? His research took him to over a dozen countries including Switzerland, Gaelic Islands, Alaska, Florida, Southern Pacific Islands, Africa, Australia, Peru and the Amazon. He examined the native people based on the health of their mouths as well as their overall physical and mental health. He photographed thousands to prove the absence of deformity and illness. He meticulously recorded their diets and took samples of food home to measure the nutrient content. He funded his research himself guaranteeing that his conclusions were free from corporate or political influence. As he accumulated data, a pattern emerged, allowing him to amass an understanding of what leads to strong dental, physical, and mental health, regardless of geographic location or genetics.

In a mountainous village of Switzerland, he found a population that had strong, straight, white teeth with less than 1% decay despite not brushing their teeth! In addition, the men were strong, the women beautiful, and there was an absence of tuberculosis, which plagued many neighboring regions at the time. Their primary source of calories was raw dairy products (milk, cheese, cream, and butter). They also readily consumed rye, sourdough (fermented) bread. They ate meat approximately once a week and rarely ate vegetables. They ritualistically prepared special, nutrient dense food (butter) to be saved for use during times of physical development like pregnancy and infancy. On a Gaelic island, he found a population in excellent health. They did not consume fruit, vegetables, or animals. Their main source of calories came from fish, seaweed, and fermented oats. They considered cod head and cod liver sacred food to be saved for pregnant women and young children. In Alaska, Dr. Price found a hardy, robust population free from dental decay or deformities, as well as diseases common to that time. The Alaskan tribes ate mostly fish, seal oil, and blubber. They had no access to plant foods or lean meats. They considered dried salmon eggs a sacred food. In Florida, Dr. Price found Indian tribes that survived on a diet of reptiles and meat. Their teeth were strong and facial bones broad. Islands in the South Pacific maintained a diet of seafood, pork, plants, coconut, fruit, taro, and fermented foods. Similarly, Dr. Price observed that the people of this tribe were also content and happy. Everywhere Dr. Price went he found the same thing. Consuming a tribal diet resulted in no tooth decay, emotional stability, good physical development, and a low to absent disease rate. All of these cultures were cut off geographically from the arrival of westernized, processed food and toothpaste!

Weston Price expanded his research to include an assessment of the tribal populations whose routes of transportation allowed them access to outside sources of food. He also studied genetically similar populations that geographically had better access to more westernized food options. Once access to outside, processed food was established (flour, condensed milk, chocolate), Dr. Price saw an increase in decay, dental deformities, tuberculosis, and infertility. The incidence of dental deformities, susceptibility to disease, and overall poor mental and physical health increased with each generation as its diet became further and further removed from its traditional tribal diet. What struck me most about Dr. Price's findings was that it didn't matter what the native tribe or village was eating, as long as the food was unprocessed. They didn't require meat from animals to build muscles. They didn't need antioxidants from cruciferous vegetables. They didn't shun saturated fats. They ate only what was available to them based on climate and geography. And yet, they had no heart disease, diabetes, cancer, or autoimmune disease. They were strong and healthy. Amazing!

The diets of healthy, non-industrialized people have much in common regardless of genetics, location, climate, or food source. As I learned at IIN and NGI, these are the characteristics of traditional food diets as determined by Dr. Price's research:

1. All traditional diets contain no refined or denatured foods like: refined sugar, white flour, high fructose corn syrup, canned foods, pasteurized, homogenized, skim or low-fat milk, refined or hydrogenated vegetable oils, protein powders, or additives and artificial colorings of any kind.
2. All traditional cultures consume food derived from animals. The source can vary greatly and include: fish, shellfish, land and sea mammals, eggs, raw milk, cheese, butter, reptiles, and insects. In every culture, the entire animal was eaten—skin, flesh, organs, bone marrow, and fat.
3. Primitive diets were nutrient dense and contained four times the minerals, water

soluble vitamins, and ten times the fat soluble vitamins as found in the modern American diet.

4. All traditional cultures consumed some cooked food and some raw food. Raw milk, for example, is full of components that strengthen the immune system. Modern pasteurization kills many of these components.

5. All non-industrialized diets included some form of fermented food that had a high content of enzymes and beneficial bacteria.

6. All nuts, seeds, and grains underwent a long soaking, sprouting, and fermenting process that allowed for a breakdown of the naturally occurring toxins and anti-nutrients that inhibit their complete digestion.

7. Traditional diets were high in fat, ranging from 30% to 80% of the diet. However, a very small percentage of that fat came from polyunsaturated fat (corn oil). The majority of the fat was saturated (butter, lard) and monounsaturated (olive oil).

8. Traditional diets contain a healthy 1:1 balance of omega 6 fats to omega 3 fats. Modern American diets have been seen to have an imbalance of omega 6 to omega 3 fats of nearly 40:1.

9. All traditional diets use some salt, however, that salt is in the form of unrefined sea salt.

10. All traditional cultures made use of animal bones, usually in the form of bone broth.
11. Traditional cultures made provisions for the health of future generations. They reserved super nutrient dense food for times of pregnancy, infancy and early childhood. They also valued passing on the principles of proper diet and nutrition to the young.

Although many of the conclusions above run contrary to my beliefs as a vegan-wannabe and contrary to the gluten free, grain free paleo world I have been trying to embrace, it's hard to ignore the obvious results. Maybe it doesn't matter if we are vegan, paleo, macrobiotic, ayurvedic, or Ben and Jerry devotees. I think what becomes apparent from Dr. Price's extensive research is that what matters most is that we avoid processed food! If native tribes in Alaska can maintain superior health while consuming a diet primarily made up of whale blubber, I think it's safe to say that heart disease is not caused by saturated fat. In fact, maybe fat is not the demon it's been made out to be after all. Maybe instead of butter and eggs, high cholesterol comes from too many cookies and white bread? It certainly makes sense to me!

"When I was five years old, my mother always told me that happiness was the key to life. When I went to school, they asked me what I wanted to be when I grew up. I wrote down 'happy'. They told me I didn't understand the assignment, and I told them they didn't understand life."

—John Lennon

CHAPTER SEVEN

AFTER YOU CLEAN THE KITCHEN

The paleo diet, as I once imagined, is not a cult of people who have shed their business clothes for loincloths. They do not shun modern society, avoid technology, or cook all their meals outdoors over open flames. They do not walk around with a wooden club in one hand and a giant drumstick in the other. Instead, they have looked at our overly processed food supply, our ever-expanding waistlines, and our skyrocketing disease rate and said, there must be a better way; and in fact, there IS a better way. For many thousands of years, food came packaged by nature, not factories, obesity was nonexistent, and we died from accidents or infection, not lifestyle diseases. What I find particularly intriguing about the paleo diet is that it is not just about the food you eat. There is so much more to the paleo philosophy that has nothing to do with food, yet so much to do with your health. If you are trying to feel better, have more energy, reverse disease, act preventatively, reach peak athletic performance, or just simply be happy and healthy, the paleo lifestyle will give you so much more than a good pot roast recipe.

EXHIBIT A: Exercise

Everyone knows that exercise is a key component to good health. It helps you to burn calories, build muscles, and keep your heart in shape. But we were built for more than just spending our requisite 30 minutes on the treadmill each day. Prior to the advent of agriculture, our ancestors did more than just hunt and gather. They spent their days walking, running, sprinting, climbing, carrying, building, playing, dancing, and relaxing. They had active lives out of necessity rather than based on a doctor's recommendation. Their movements were functional and purposeful. With each technological advance, we have discovered a way to eliminate movement from nearly every aspect of our lives. So much so that we now have to schedule exercise into our day. There are many primal activities still available to us despite technology including walking the dog, chasing our kids, swimming, walking to town, splitting wood, planting a garden, shoveling snow, pulling weeds, and cleaning the house. These activities are functional, purposeful, and sometimes fun! They keep us strong, flexible, and they don't require a gym membership. Don't get me wrong. I belong to a gym and try to get there most days of the week. But since learning about the paleo philosophy, I have started to change the way I look at my exercise routine. Instead of looking to log time, miles, and calorie burn on an aerobic machine, I have started to lean more towards heavy lifting, functional training, and aerobic activities that make me happy in addition to making me sweat (yay Zumba)! I make sure I stretch, strengthen my core, and make variety a priority. I consider walking the dog a privilege rather than a chore. But the most important thing I have learned from the paleo exercise philosophy is to rest. Primal humans had intense bouts of energy expenditure. When they weren't running for their lives, building shelter, or moving a boulder, they rested. I used to think that in order to be healthy I had to get to the gym for an hour every day. But now I understand that my DNA, my genetic code that is largely unchanged from my primal self, expects short difficult bouts of energy, continuous daily movement, and periods of rest and recovery. On Sundays when I sleep in a bit, go to church, do some laundry, make dinner, and snuggle on the couch with my family, I am contributing to my health just as much as taking a killer spin class. I think, in our society, we feel like we have to be really sick, or attending a funeral, to take a day off. If you give yourself permission to exercise for good health then you also must give yourself permission to rest for good health. If you don't, illness or injury will certainly step in and force the break for you.

EXHIBIT B: Sleep

For millions of years, humans rose in the morning when light from the sun alerted them to the new day and began to wind down, rest, and sleep when the sun went down. Our brains recognized sunrise as the time to release hormones that perk us up and give us energy for the day to come. Similarly, in the evening, sunset triggers our brains to release different hormones that create a state of relaxation to help us transition into sleep. This pattern of natural wake and sleep, dictated by light and dark, is called our circadian rhythm. Our modern society has moved us so far away from this natural pattern of waking and sleeping with the sun by giving us the power to create the appearance of daylight twenty four hours a day. I am not suggesting that people who follow a paleo lifestyle have gotten rid of their alarm clocks and told their bosses they need to be home before sunset, lest they turn into a werewolf. But they have taken a look at the dramatic turn we have taken away from natural sleep cycles and what affects it has had on our health.

In *The Primal Blueprint*, Mark Sisson explains in detail the significant repercussions of living a life contrary to our circadian rhythm. Sleep deprivation, as we all know, makes us impatient and cranky at times. But its affects run much deeper than simply making us feel and act tired. Lack of sleep can influence concentration and memory retention, increase blood pressure and the risk for heart disease, and increase inflammation while decreasing immune function. It also increases stress hormones and messes with the hormones that control your appetite. As a result, sleep deprivation has been linked to weight gain and an increased risk of obesity, heart disease, and inflammatory diseases. Losing sleep interferes with fat burning, muscle building, and cellular repair and regeneration. In other words, if you skimp on sleep, you undermine your body's ability to reap the benefits from your efforts to eat healthy and exercise.

I know it is impossible to schedule ourselves around the rising and the setting of the sun. But when you begin to look at sleep through a paleo lens, you may start to see how really off you are from what your DNA is still programed to expect. There are many paleo recommendations when it comes to getting enough sleep.

- Expose your skin to at least fifteen minutes of natural sunlight every day. Sunlight provides the most concentrated form of vitamin D which decreases stress hormones and helps decrease your risk for cancer.

- Before going to sleep, avoid strenuous exercise, a large meal, alcohol, artificial light, stress, and caffeine. (Good luck with that one!)

- Create a relaxing bedtime ritual: drink warm tea, take a warm bath, use aromatherapy oils, read for pleasure instead of work, listen to soothing music, meditate, pray; whatever works best for you.

- Create an environment conducive to a sound sleep. Your room should be quiet, cool, and totally dark. Your skin absorbs light just like your eyes do. So consider black out curtains, not just an eye mask.

- Avoid artificial light before bed. This includes computers, TV, cell phones, digital alarm clocks, and nightlights.

- Consider using a light alarm. This type of alarm gets gradually brighter for a length of time that you set, allowing you to wake from light rather than sound. You can also have it play music that gets gradually louder while you get used to the light.

- Strive to keep a regular bedtime and wake time whenever possible.

- Strive for eight to nine hours every night. (If you have autoimmune disease, ten to thirteen hours are recommended!)

- If you have autoimmune disease, sleep must become a priority. The more you sleep, the more your body has time to heal.

- If you can't get enough sleep at night, consider taking a short nap during the day. Twenty to thirty minutes have been shown to decrease inflammation.

It is much easier for me to make a list of what you should do. I know it seems impossible to fit one more thing into your day. I get it! I am trying to do it too. Prior to my cancer diagnosis, I spent four years sleeping sitting up in bed because of the pain in my hips and spine. I didn't yet know I had ankylosing spondylitis. Those four years came during and after the birth of my three kids. So essentially, I had spent six years up half the night with infants plus four years sitting up in bed. That's a decade of no sleep! I wonder now how many of those years contributed to my autoimmune issues and cancer diagnosis. Of course there was nothing I could do at that time to change the fact that I had to feed crying babies in the middle of the night and that I was too uncomfortable to lie down. But

After You Clean The Kitchen **101**

with my paleo education, I now realize how important sleep is. I try my best to be sleeping every night by ten and my alarm wakes me at six every morning. I point the digital alarm numbers away from my face. I haven't started using a light alarm because I don't think my husband would appreciate a full sunrise in our bedroom on the days he gets to sleep in. My sister, however, is using a light alarm and feels more rested and energetic than when she was blasted awake by her old alarm. Did I mention how much my husband snores? Make that two decades of no sleep! I wear earplugs at night to block out the snoring, not entirely effective but better than nothing, and I don't have infants anymore so I don't have to worry about needing to hear if they are crying. They are all old enough to walk into my room and wake me up to tell me they puked. Can't they just tell me in the morning? Before tucking in, I spend at least fifteen minutes saying prayers and writing in my gratitude journal. Find what you can work into your schedule and make the quality and quantity of your sleep a priority. Just like with food, these recommendations are not an all or nothing proposition. Every choice you make to get more, and better quality sleep makes a difference in your goal towards good health.

EXHIBIT 3: Stress

I saved stress for last because it's a doozy! Since my

cancer diagnosis, I have had countless doctors tell me I need to reduce my stress level. I just about laughed in their faces. Three kids, (in grammar school, high school, and college), cancer, autoimmune disease, fifty thousand doctor appointments, fifty thousand dollars in medical bills...how, exactly, am I supposed to reduce my stress? Meditation, they said. I tried that. I felt stressed spending so much time trying to relax! So, for a dozen years, my stress levels continued to grow to gargantuan proportions. I felt that I was doing everything I could to address what I had control over—food. But stress, I believed, was out of my hands.

Once again, paleo stepped in to open my eyes to the difference between modern stress and ancient stress. Our bodies are truly remarkable in all that they do for us. Stress, to a certain degree, is a good thing. For as long as humans have roamed the earth, stress has been a life saving asset. When we are threatened, our brains set off the emergency alarm and produce stress hormones (cortisol and adrenaline) that allow our bodies to focus on the danger at hand. These hormones rise quickly, decrease less important bodily functions, and increase our strength and energy for a short period of time. This burst allows us to fight, sprint, and essentially survive. Once the danger has passed, hormones quickly reduce and the alarm is reset to the off position. Enter modern life. Unlike the occasional encounter with a man-eating beast in the woods, modern stressors are insidious and relentless. Long frustrating commutes, road rage, work deadlines, bills, illness, school bullies, college applications, more bills, junk food, Ebola, horrible bosses, terrorists, broken appliances, the rainbow wheelie on your computer, more bills, sleep deprivation...the list is endless. Now, instead of having infrequent, yet life threatening stressors, we live in a world where we experience never ending levels of stress. The emergency alarm switch in our brain stays in the on position. Here's the problem. Our DNA does not know the difference between a bear in the woods and a speeding ticket. To our brain, stress is stress, and cortisol is released. Our bodies are not equipped to handle constant levels of cortisol streaming through our system, day after day, commute after commute, and fast food meal after fast food meal.

Through visits to the Blum Center, *The Paleo Approach* by Sarah Ballantyne, and countless other paleo books, I have come to have a deeper understanding of the role of chronic stress and disease. In a normal person, without chronic stress (does anyone fit that criteria?), cortisol peaks in the early morning then slowly decreases throughout the day, reaching its low point in the evening, at bedtime. Low cortisol before waking is important for memory retention. So that's why I can't remember why I walked up the stairs! The peak in cortisol upon waking allows you to be alert and energized in the morning and regulates bodily functions throughout the day. As your cortisol levels slowly return to their low in the evening, your body gets ready for relaxation and sleep. Or, so I was told. At the Blum Center, I actually had my cortisol levels measured. I spit into a vial every couple of hours and logged my spit schedule for the lab. The lab then graphed my cortisol levels in comparison to the normal levels expected. Guess what? My cortisol was high all day and night! My levels dipped slightly in the afternoon which was giving me the sensation that I needed a cup of coffee and a candy bar, PRONTO, or I just couldn't go on. Another common, but abnormal, pattern is to maintain a moderate level of elevated cortisol all day, with a coffee/candy bar slump at 3:00, and an inconvenient "second wind" close to bedtime. This pattern is what the experts call "tired and wired". You muddle through your day, crash at 3:00pm, have enough energy at 9:00pm to watch three episodes of NCIS, and then lay in bed all night, tired, but unable to fall asleep. Any of this sound familiar? The stress and frustration we feel by not being able to fall or stay asleep just adds more cortisol to an already bubbling cauldron.

I didn't need a crash course on cortisol to teach me about the physical or emotional stresses so prevalent in today's society. I can rattle them off in my not-so-good-sleep:

- Physical stressors: injury, illness, dehydration, hunger, fasting (yes, a juice cleanse can be perceived as stress), medication, processed food, exercise, sleep deprivation, pain, discomfort...

- Emotional stressors: anxiety, fear, anger, frustration, grief, loneliness, insecurity, being overwhelmed...

Remember, what our brain perceives when we are sick, hungry, malnourished, tired, anxious, overwhelmed, scared, is – DANGER! – release cortisol to increase survival. What happens next in our body is amazing, life saving stuff, especially back in the caveman day. When cortisol is released, our body uses laser sharp focus to release stored glucose and send it directly to our brain and muscles. This quick fuel allows us to think sharply and run for our lives! At the same time, it shuts down any process considered non-essential for immediate survival. Such non-essentials include digestion, reproduction, growth, immunity, collagen formation, protein synthesis, and bone formation. Quite efficient for a caveman, but utterly disastrous for us. Chronically elevated cortisol causes a breakdown of muscle tissue, increased food cravings, insulin resistance, mood disorders, impaired memory, abdominal fat, susceptibility to infection, and the killer for me...leaky gut and inflammation! I am beginning to think EVERYTHING causes leaky gut! The end result is this. Chronic stress increases your risk for autoimmune disease, heart disease, diabetes, osteoporosis, depression, infection, and cancer.

At this point on my learning curve I began to think that micromanaging everything I put in my mouth was not going to be the only answer to my poor health. I had been poo-pooing my doctor's advice to decrease stress as an impossible task for a dozen years. But after seeing my completely dysfunctional spit graph, I realized I had more issues on my plate than just gluten. After I stressed out about being so stressed out, I started to take stock of all the stressors in my life. That list, my friends, is a topic for another book. I tried very hard to convince myself that I was no longer allowed to get injured, sleep deprived, angry, frustrated, and the like. Physical and emotional feelings were out of the question if I were going to get better. Well, that strategy lasted a couple of hours. But gradually, VERY gradually, I began to realize that there were some things that I could control. I have learned to say, "no." I am very picky about the volunteer work I commit to now. I have a small group of friends and have eliminated most "obligatory" friendships. I exercise differently, more paleo. I try to keep a regular sleep and eating schedule. I attend mass daily and thank the Lord for all the blessings in my life. And, my favorite stress reducing strategy of all time, I get a weekly massage. There are many proven stress reducing tools out there—meditation, deep breathing, hobbies, time spent enjoying nature, laughter, yoga, tai chi, and aromatherapy. It is true that stress may very well be the most insidious poison of our modern day society. Don't wait until you are so sick that you are forced to remove yourself from your daily routine. Try different things and incorporate into your life what works best for you. Say, "no." Breathe. Make time for a walk. Laugh. Be grateful. Life is too short not to.

"As you grow older, you will discover that you have two hands, one for helping yourself and the other for helping others."

—Sam Levenson

CHAPTER EIGHT

BACKINTIME KITCHEN

Martine. That's the name of my amazing, gifted, intelligent, compassionate, and wonderful business partner. About seven years ago, when I was charging full steam ahead into veganism, I happened upon a small coffee shop in Mendham, New Jersey. It was a cozy, inviting space that calls you in for a warm cup of tea, lunch, and a break from the busyness of life. Sprawled on the floor, chalk in hand, was a beautiful, dark haired woman artfully inscribing the daily specials. Faster than she could fill the blackboard, my mouth was watering. Carrot-ginger soup. Sweet potato hummus. Open faced broccoli rabe sandwiches. Yum, yum, and YUM! Everything was vegan or vegetarian. I fell in love with the place. But more importantly, the dark haired woman, was Martine. I wouldn't say that I am introverted, but definitely very shy. I rarely talk to strangers but I enjoy listening to other people talk.

I am certainly not the person at a dinner party that carries the conversation with my quick wit. However, something came over me at that coffee shop that compelled me to sit next to Martine and pepper her with questions: How long have you been working here? Are you vegan or vegetarian? Do you serve breakfast, lunch, and dinner—or just lunch? And the obvious next question...will you hire me? There was something about Martine that made me want to be her best friend immediately. Within our first conversation, I learned that she had two daughters, a husband who rode a motorcycle, French parents, a passion for sustainability, and rheumatoid arthritis. Wow, I had never met another person my age with an autoimmune disease. When I go to the doctor I am the youngest person in the waiting room by at least thirty years. Martine and I had so much in common it must have been destiny for us to meet.

I was desperate to learn how to cook vegan and vegetarian fare that even my carnivorous family would want to eat. So the next day I returned ready to peel, chop, and blend whatever was put in front of me. On day two, Martine informed me that she and Judy, her chef partner, were going into New York City to do some field research. I was to stay at the shop and cook, from scratch, carrot ginger soup. They gave me a quick tutorial and off they went. OMG! I definitely should have mentioned that I didn't know how to cook! I spent the next several hours peeling mountains of carrots and chopping fresh ginger root (which I had never seen before in my life). Peel, chop, boil, and then purée in the Cuisinart. Before I knew it, it was time for me to leave and go pick my kids up from school. Fifty pots filled the sink, and the kitchen looked like an orange bomb had exploded inside. But I did manage to produce several gallons of carrot ginger soup. I fully expected to be fired the next day, if not for the taste of the soup, then certainly for the mess I left behind. Instead, Martine and Judy graciously praised my efforts, and I fell comfortably into a routine of dropping my kids at school and driving to Mendham to chop away the day. My favorite part came on Sundays when we sold our prepared food at the farmer's markets. I learned so much from Martine and Judy about cooking techniques, composting, and sustainability. Even though the coffee shop closed down a year or two later, I still have daydreams of attending culinary school, a passion sparked by my time cooking with Martine and Judy.

Fast forward seven years when I happened to bump into Martine while having lunch with some friends. We hugged for ten minutes and then promptly made plans to meet for lunch the following week. We met on Wednesday of the next week at Legal Seafood. As

I waited, gluten free menu in hand, I wondered what Martine would think about my crossover from vegan to paleo. I knew she also suffered from autoimmune diseases but had no idea where her journey had taken her in the past several years. She arrived, opened the menu, and announced "I am eating paleo now". My jaw dropped. We spent the next couple of hours catching up on kids, husbands, life, and how we both came to learn about the connection between autoimmune disease and the paleo lifestyle. Amazingly, Martine, like my sister, was able to wean off of her rheumatoid arthritis medication after going paleo. Once again, I felt destiny had brought us together.

The week after our lunch was when I attended The Natural Gourmet Institute for my paleo intensive cooking class. I spent most of my train ride home each day texting Martine about what I had learned. Immediately we knew we wanted to go into business together and incorporate our collective knowledge into producing a product that could help other people with autoimmune disease (and healthy folks too). And just like that, the concept of BackInTime Kitchen was born. Our first product, we thought, should be nourishing bone broth to sell at our local farmer's market. With that product, we hoped to attract clients to whom I could provide health coaching and Martine could provide cooking classes.

We both knew there were thousands of people out there suffering from autoimmune disease who had no idea there were answers that could help them move towards a happier and healthier life. Our target market was anyone suffering from disease (cancer, autoimmune, or otherwise), or those living in a state of general poor health due to the cumulative effects of the Standard American Diet and our overstressed, sleep deprived, modern way of living (so, basically everyone else). We knew we not only had the knowledge, but we had the compassion to help others because of our own personal stories. We also felt strongly that there must be lots of vegan/vegetarians who need to consider eating paleo because of their health. This is not an easy transition to make so one of our business goals was to create a cookbook that bridges the gap between being vegan and being paleo. Paleo-Vegan Yum!

I included this chapter not to tell you all about my business aspirations or to give you the top ten tips to business success. There are many books out there that can do a far better job at that than I can. Instead, I want you to know, learn, understand, and embrace this one thing. You can do it too! I have spent the past dozen years either being sick or waiting to get sick again. I stopped volunteering at my kid's schools, stopped inviting groups of friends over for dinner, and gave up hopes of ever having a real career again. Basically, I was living in fear. I was afraid that if I did any of those things, and I got sick again, that I would let someone down. Every time I felt well for a period of time, I would start to regain hope that I might finally be healthy. But over and over again, I would be healthy and hopeful one day, and then find myself in pain, or with fevers, or with Crohn's attacks that would last for six months. I began to doubt every healthy lifestyle decision I had made. Why bother exercising and avoiding fast food if I was just going to be sick anyway?

The good (no, great!) news is that I don't feel that way any more. Everything I have learned about the causes of leaky gut and how it leads to autoimmune disease has put everything in perspective. I now can see why my seemingly "healthy whole grain" diet was undermining my health all along. Even on days that I don't feel great, I don't automatically assume that it is the beginning of my next downward spiral. And the best part is, I have proof that the paleo principals I have adopted are working, no matter how I feel. By eliminating gluten, grains, beans, and dairy, I have kept my inflammatory markers (C-reactive protein) in check. In fact, I have not had any relapse of any kind since adopting a paleo-vegan lifestyle. That doesn't mean my health is going to be perfect from now on.

I know I have a long way to go to fully heal my gut, work to reduce stressors in my life, and eliminate environmental toxins. But I am confident that I am on the right path and I no longer live in fear of becoming ill again. If I do get sick, I know what diet tweaks I need to make. I know to get a little extra sleep. I know to focus on stress reduction. I am confident that I can stay on my path to wellness. I have been liberated from the fear that had caged me for so many years. And I know that this liberation is possible for you too! I don't know the first thing about starting a business. If you told me a year ago that I was going to be writing a book and starting a business, I would have thought you were crazy. If you are a little sick, or very sick, I want you to know that illness does not have to be a life sentence. You do not have to live in fear. You can reclaim your health, take on your passion, and really live again! For me, it's BackInTime Kitchen. What is it going to be for you?

"Clouds come floating into my life, no longer to carry rain or usher storm, but to add color to my sunset sky."

—Rabindranath Tagore

CHAPTER NINE

THE BEGINNING

I LOVE food. I'm obsessed with it, actually. I could not spend a single day as a paleo-vegan if I lost my ability to do my happy dance when I eat something awesome. Even if it meant I would feel better. But you CAN have it all. You can feel better and eat amazing food, without guilt, deprivation, or dieting! You can make small changes one at a time, or jump in with two feet right away. If you are tired of having headaches, low energy, ten pounds that refuse to budge, skin rashes, insomnia, low libido, thyroid issues, anxiety, aches and pains, a bloated belly, brain fog, or full blown autoimmune disease, you can do something about it! Here's what you can do, right now, to begin your journey towards feeling better every day.

1. Upgrade the quality of your food.
   If you eat meat, make sure it is 100% grass

fed and grass finished. Buy free range, cage free, organic chicken and wild fish.

When you can afford it, buy organic fruits and vegetables.

Eat local and in-season.

Swap iodized table salt for unrefined sea salt.

2. Do an elimination diet to see what foods you might be sensitive to.

   I recommend *The Virgin Diet* by J.J. Virgin.

   If this sounds overwhelming to you, start by giving up gluten for one month and see how you feel.

3. Don't be afraid to eat fat and change which fats you are eating.

   Use coconut oil, ghee (butter without milk solids), avocados, and olive oil.

   Avoid all processed vegetable oils like corn oil, canola oil, sunflower oil, soybean oil, and safflower oil.

4. Avoid processed foods and sugar as much as possible.

5. Try incorporating bone broth and fermented foods into your diet.

6. Exercise like a caveman.

   Move often, lift heavy, have fun.

7. Sleep eight or more hours a night.

   Make your room dark, cool, and quiet.

   Give yourself time before bed without electronics or TV.

8. Get out in the sun everyday.
9. Find a way to decrease your daily stress. Practice gratitude, pray, get massages, or whatever works for you.
10. If you have autoimmune disease, follow the Autoimmune Protocol.
For details, read *The Paleo Approach* by Sarah Ballantyne.
11. Visit www.functionalmedicine.org to find a functional medicine doctor in your area.
12. BELIEVE that you can feel better than you do right now!

So, my story begins. With BackInTime Kitchen and Paleo-Vegan Yum, I am ready to hit the ground running toward endless possibilities and leave my fear of illness in the dust. No matter your age, diagnosis, budget, or overall health, it is never too late to make positive changes in your life. Why not make this your beginning too? Come on. It will be fun!

"Live as if you were to die tomorrow. Learn as if you were to live forever."

—Mahatma Gandhi

— MY FAVORITES —

BEST PALEO BOOK (for science geeks)
The Paleo Approach by Sarah Ballantyne

BEST PALEO BOOK (for non-science geeks)
It Starts With Food by Dallas and Melissa Hartwig

BEST PALEO COOKBOOK/ WEBSITE/BLOG
NomNomPaleo: Food for Humans by Michelle Tam and Henry Fong

BEST VEGAN COOKBOOK/ WEBSITE/BLOG
YumUniverse

BEST GENERAL HEALTH WEBSITE/BLOG
Mind, Body, Green

BEST ELIMINATION DIET
The Virgin Diet by J.J. Virgin

BEST BOOKS LINKING POOR DIET TO ILLNESS
Nutrition and Physial Degeneration by Weston A. Price, MD

The China Study by T. Colin Campbell, MD

Grain Brain by David Perlmutter, MD

BEST CANCER COOKBOOK

One Bite at a Time: Nourishing Recipes for Cancer Survivors and their Friends by Rebecca Katz

BEST BOOK ABOUT EMOTIONAL EATING

Women, Food, and God: An Unexpected Path to Almost Everything by Geneen Roth

BEST VEGAN MAGAZINE

VegNews

BEST PALEO MAGAZINE

Paleo Magazine

BEST FAMILY FRIENDLY DOCUMENTARY ABOUT THE HEALING POWER OF FOOD

Fat, Sick and Nearly Dead

BEST DOCUMENTARY ABOUT TRYING A VEGAN LIFESTYLE

Vegucated

BEST DOCUMENTARY ABOUT ALTERNATIVE CANCER THERAPIES

The Gerson Miracle

"Do not read, as children do, to amuse yourself, or like the ambitious, for the purpose of instruction. No, read in order to live."

—Gustave Flaubert

—— RESOURCES ——

PALEO BOOKS

It Starts With Food by Dallas and Melissa Hartwig

The Primal Blueprint by Mark Sisson

Primal Body, Primal Mind: Beyond the Paleo Diet for Total Health and a Longer Life by Nora T. Gedgaudas, CNS, CNT

Your Personal Paleo Code: The 3-Step Plan to Lose Weight, Reverse Disease, and Stay Fit and Healthy for Life by Chris Kresser

The Paleo Dieters Missing Link by Adam Farrah, BS

The Paleo Approach: Reverse Autoimmune Disease and Heal Your Gut by Sarah Ballantyne, PhD

Practical Paleo: A Customized Approach to Health and a Whole Foods Lifestyle by Diane Sanfilippo, BS, NC

Eat the Yolks: Discover Paleo, Fight Food Lies, and Reclaim Your Health by Liz Wolfe, NTP

The Paleo Solution: The Original Human Diet by Robb Wolf

The Paleo Diet by Loren Cordain, PhD

VEGAN BOOKS

The Engine 2 Diet by Rip Esselstyn

Prevent and Reverse Heart Disease: The Revolutionary, Scientifically Proven Nutrition Based Cure by Caldwell B. Esselstyn, Jr., MD

Forks Over Knives: The Plant Based Way to Health edited by Gene Stone

Crazy, Sexy, Cancer by Kris Carr

Crazy, Sexy, Diet: Eat Your Veggies, Ignite Your Spark, and Live Like You Meant It! by Kris Carr

The China Study: Startling Implications for Diet, Weight Loss and Long-Term Health by T. Colin Campbell, PhD and Thomas M. Campbell II

Power Vegan: Plant-Fueled Nutrition for Maximum Health and Fitness by Rea Frey

Vegan Bodybuilding and Fitness: The Complete Guide to Building Your Body on a Plant Based Diet by Robert Cheeke

GENERAL HEALTH BOOKS

The Virgin Diet by J.J. Virgin

Digestive Health with Real Food by Agalee Jacob, MS, RD

Year of No Sugar: A Memoir by Eve O. Schaub

100 Days of Real Food: How We Did It, What We Learned, and 100 Easy, Wholesome Recipes Your Family Will Love by Lisa Leake

Candida Albicans: Could Yeast Be Your Problem? by Leon Chaitow, DO, ND

The Immune System Recovery Plan by Susan Blum, MD, MPH

The Complete Low-FODMAP Diet: A Revolutionary Plan for Managing IBS and Other Digestive Disorders by Sue Shepherd, PhD. and Peter Gibson, MD

Integrative Nutrition by Joshua Rosenthal

The Gerson Therapy: The Proven Nutritional Program for Cancer and Other Illnesses by Charlotte Gerson and Morton Walker, DPM

Nourishing Traditions by Sally Fallon

Grain Brain: The Surprising Truth about Wheat, Carbs, and Sugar—Your Brain's Silent Killers by David Perlmutter, MD

The Blood Sugar Solution: The Ultrahealthy Program for Losing Weight, Preventing Disease and Feeling Great Now! by Mark Hyman, MD

Wheat Belly by William Davis, MD

21 Day Sugar Detox by Diane Sanfilippo, BS, NC

The World According to Monsanto: Pollution, Corruption and the Control of Our Food Supply. An Investigation into the World's Most Controversial Company by Marie-Monique Robin

The Wisdom and Healing Power of Whole Foods: The Ultimate Handbook for Using Whole Foods and Lifestyle Changes to Bolster Your Body's Ability to Repair and Regulate Itself by Patrick Quillin, PhD, RD, CNS

The Food Revolution. How Your Diet Can Help Save Your Life and the World by John Robbins

Pandora's Lunchbox: How Processed Food took Over the American Meal by Melanie Warner

Breaking the Vicious Cycle: Intestinal Health through Diet by Elaine Gottschall, BS, MSc

The Body Ecology Diet: Recovering Your Health and Rebuilding Your Immunity by Donna Gates.

Patient Heal Thyself by Jordon Rubin, NMD, PhD

The Inflammation Free Diet Plan by Monica Reinagel

Whitewash: The Disturbing Truth about Cow's Milk and Your Health by Joseph Keon

Food and Healing: How What You Eat Determines Your Health, Your Wellbeing, and the Quality of Your Life by AnneMarie Colbin

Ultraprevention: The 6-Week Plan That Will Make You Healthy For Life by Mark Hyman, MD

Ultra-Longevity: The 7-Step Program For Younger, Healthier You by Mark Hyman, MD

Clean: Remove, Restore, Rejuvenate. The Revolutionary Program to Restore the Body's Natural Ability to Heal Itself by Alejandro Junger, MD

Food Rules: An Eater's Manual by Michael Pollan

Women, Food and God: An Unexpected Path to Almost Everything by Geneen Roth

When You Eat at the Refrigerator Pull Up a Chair: 50 Ways to Feel Thin, Gorgeous, and Happy (When You Feel Anything But) by Geneen Roth

Eat to Live: The Revolutionary Formula for Fast and Sustained Weight Loss by Joel Fuhrman, MD

Super Immunity: The Essential Nutrition Guide for Boosting Your Body's Defenses to Live Longer, Stronger, and Disease Free by Joel Fuhrman, MD

PALEO COOKBOOKS

The Paleo Approach Cookbook by Sarah Ballantyne, PhD

Practical Paleo by Dianne Sanfillippo, BS. NC

The Paleo Diet Cookbook by Loren Cordain, PhD

The Autoimmune Paleo Cookbook by Mickey Trescott, NTP

Paleo Slow Cooking: Over 140 Practical, Primal, Whole Food Recipes for the Slow Cooker by Dominique DeVito

NomNom Paleo: Food for Humans by Michelle Tam and Henry Fong

The 30 Day Guide to Paleo Cooking by Haley Mason and Bill Staley

Everyday Paleo Thai Cuisine by Sarah Fragaso

Against All Grain: Delectable Paleo Recipes to Eat Well and Feel Great by Danielle Walker

Make It Paleo by Haley Mason and Bill Staley

Powerful Paleo Superfoods: The Best Primal-Friendly Foods for Burning Fat, Building Muscle, and Optimal Health by Heather Connell, RHNC

The Paleo Kitchen: Finding Primal Joy In Modern Cooking by Juli Bauer and George Bryant

Paleo-Vegan Smoothies by Sadia Sandeela

Paleo Magazine: Reader's Favorite Cookbook. Favorite Paleo, Primal and Grain Free Recipes

Paleo Magazine: Reader's Favorite Holiday Recipes. All Paleo, Primal, and Grain Free

VEGAN COOKBOOKS

Clean Food: A Seasonal Guide to Eating Close to the Source by Terry Walters

Pretty Delicious by Candice Kumai

Chloe's Kitchen: 125 Easy Delicious Recipes for Making the Food You Love the Vegan Way by Chloe Coscarelli

Crazy, Sexy, Kitchen: 150 Plant-Empowered Recipes to Ignite a Mouthwatering Revolution by Kris Carr, with Chef Chad Sarno

Paleo-Vegan Smoothies by Sadia Sandeela

Liquid Raw. Over 125 Juices, Smoothies, Soups, and Other Raw Beverages by Lisa Montgomery

The Conscious Cook: Delicious Meatless Recipes That Will Change the Way You Eat by Tal Ronnen

Vegan Vittles by Jo Stepaniak

The Candle Café Cookbook: More Than 150 Enlightened Recipes from New Yorks Renowned Vegan Restaurant by Joy Pierson and Bart Potenza

Vegan Cooking For Carnivores: Over 125 Recipes So Tasty You Won't Miss the Meat by Roberto Martin

The Blender Girl: 100 Gluten-Free Vegan Recipes by Tess Masters

GENERAL HEALTH COOKBOOKS

Digestive Health with Real Food: The Cookbook by Aglaee Jacob, MS, RD

The Grain Brain Cookbook by David Perlmutter, MD

The Autoimmune Paleo Cookbook by Mickey Trescott, NTP

Wheat Belly Cookbook by William Davis, MD

One Bite at a Time: Nourishing Recipes for Cancer Survivors and Their Friends by Rebecca Katz

Cooking With Coconut Oil: Gluten-Free, Grain-Free Recipes for Good Living by Elizabeth Nyland

Fast, Fresh and Green: More Than 90 Delicious Recipes for Veggie Lovers by Susie Middletown

Eat Fresh Food: Awesome Recipes for Teen Chefs by Rozanne Gold

500 of the Healthiest Recipes and Health Tips You'll Ever Need by Hazel Courtney and Stephen Langley

Superfoods: The Food and Medicine of the Future by David Wolfe

The Greens Cookbook by Deborah Madison

Greens Glorious Greens: More Than 140 Ways to Prepare All Those Great-Tasting, Super-Healthy, Beautiful Leafy Greens by Johnna Albl and Catherine Walthers

The Longevity Kitchen: Satisfying, Big Flavor Recipes Featuring the Top 16 Age-Busting Power Foods by Rebecca Katz and Mat Edelson

Allergy-Friendly Food for Families: 120 Gluten-Free, Dairy-Free, Nut-Free, Egg-Free and Soy-Free Recipes Everyone Will Love from the Editors of KIWI

New Vegetarian Cooking: 120 Fast, Fresh and Fabulous Recipes by Rose Elliot

The Mayo Clinic William-Sonoma Cookbook: Simple Solutions for Eating Well

The Healthy Kitchen: Recipes for a Better Body, Life and Spirit by Andrew Weil, MD and Rosie Daley

MAGAZINES

VegNews

Vegetarian Times

Paleo Magazine

Living Without (Gluten Free and Dairy Free)

Clean Eating

Life Extension Magazine

Natural Health

Simply Gluten Free

On Fitness

Oxygen

Well Being Journal

FILMS

Food Matters

Hungry for Change

Fat, Sick, and Nearly Dead

The Gerson Miracle

Vegucated

Forks Over Knives

Fast Food Nation

Supersize Me

Crazy, Sexy, Cancer

Food, Inc.

WORKS CITED

Ballantyne, Sarah. *The Paleo Approach: Reverse Autoimmune Disease and Heal Your Body.* Victory Belt Publishing, 2013. Print.

Campbell, T. Colin, and Thomas M. Campbell. *The China Study: The Most Comprehensive Study of Nutrition Ever Conducted and the Startling Implications for Diet, Weight Loss and Long-Term Health.* Dallas, TX: BenBella, 2005. Print.

Fallon, Sally. "Traditional Foods." Institute For Integrative Nutrition. New York, New York. 17 Oct. 2009. Lecture.

Farrah, Adam. *The Paleo Dieter's Missing Link.* Paleo Media Group, 2013. Print.

Forks Over Knives | The Film. Dir. Lee Fulkerson. Monica Beach Media, 2011. Film.

Gerson, Charlotte, and Morton Walker. *The Gerson Therapy: The Proven Nutritional Program for Cancer and Other Illnesses.* New York: Kensington, 2006. Print.

Hartwig, Dallas, and Melissa Hartwig. *It Starts with Food.* Las Vegas: Victory Belt Publishing, 2012. Print.

Price, Weston A., DDS. *Nutrition and Physical Degeneration.* Price-Pottenger Nutrition Foundation, 2008. Print.

Ravage, Barbara. *The GI Handbook: How the Glycemic Index Works.* Hauppauge, NY: Barrons Educational Series, 2005. Print.

Sanfilippo, Diane. *The 21 Day Sugar Detox: Bust Sugar & Carb Cravings Naturally.* Tuttle Publishing, 2013. Print.

Sisson, Mark. *The Primal Blueprint.* Malibu, CA: Primal Nutrition, 2009. Print.

Vegucated. Dir. Marisa Miller Wolfson. Kind Green Planet, 2010. Film.

Virgin, JJ. *The Virgin Diet: Drop 7 Foods, Lose 7 Pounds, Just 7 Days.* Don Mills, Ontario: Harlequin, 2012. Print.

"For Attractive lips, speak words of
kindness.
For lovely eyes, seek out the good
in people.
For a slim figure, share your food
with the hungry.
For beautiful hair, let a child run
their fingers through it once
a day.
For poise, walk with the knowledge
that you never walk alone."

—Sam Levenson

SO GRATEFUL

For my husband, Kevin, who has supported me physically, emotionally, and financially, through all the craziness that chronic illness brings to a marriage.

For my kids, Erin, Keith, and John. Thank you for allowing me to subject you to all my ideas and recipes, and for picking up the slack when I was a part time mom. I love you!

For my mom and dad, Tom and Elvira. You gave me the one and only thing I ever needed to survive—unconditional love.

For my in-laws, Pat and Allan. Thank you for the endless hours of babysitting, support and prayers.

For Aunt Gerry and Uncle Dave. Thank you for dropping everything whenever I needed you—and for the back rubs. ☺

For my sister, Marylou. Thank you for believing in my ideas about autoimmune disease, jumping in with two feet, and supporting me along the way.

For my brother David and sista Retzel. I am so grateful for the example you set with your lives and for holding me up in prayer.

For my sister, Trish. Laughter is the best medicine and you are hilarious!

For my sister-in-law, Colleen. Thank you for loving my kids (and dog!) as much as I do.

For all my nieces and nephews: Tom, Dave, Caitlin, Peter, Craig, Mason, Jonah, Clare, Toby, Joshua, Bernadette, and Francis. I am so blessed to have such a great family!

For Dave Domino. For designing my book cover!

For all my many friends and families: The Campbells, Shumakers, Dominos, Sodustas, Zalameas, and Fabers. And for Precisely Right (Sue and Lori), St. Vincent Martyr, Villa Walsh, Oratory Prep, and Madison High. I know I am always in your prayers.

For Eileen Fischetti. For your healing touch during our massage sessions.

For Martine, my partner and friend. This is just the beginning...

For Lisa, my accountability partner and friend. I could not have done it without you!

For Becky. Thank you for your prayers and friendship.

For Catherine. We have laughed and cried over ten thousand lunches at SoHo 33. There is nothing that can't be made better by a good friend and good food!

For Cathy, my BB, for always being there.

For The Blum Center Staff. For helping me find answers to questions I didn't even know to ask and for introducing me to the wonderful world of functional medicine.

For my oncologist, Dr. Michaelson, who made me laugh when I wanted to cry.

For my rheumatologist, Dr. Rosenstein, who never made my questions sound stupid.

For Steve and Agnes. Thank you for giving my life meaning and including me in your rosary chain.

For my God, who has given me immeasurable blessings.

And last, but not least:

For Andrew, my AWESOME trainer, who made me write this book!

"And in the end, it is not the years in your life that count. It's the life in your years."

—Abraham Lincoln